MUSCLE BUILDING

(ORIGINAL VERSION, RESTORED)

By

EARLE LIEDERMAN

America's Leading Director of Physical Education

Originally Published in 1924

PUBLISHED BY O'Faolain Patriot LLC, Copyright 2011
info@PhysicalCultureBooks.com
Published in the United States of America

ISBN-13: 978-1466442757

ISBN-10: 1466442751

To Order More Copies Visit: Physical Culture Books.com

TABLE OF CONTENTS

PREFACE

IT may interest the reader to know that the manuscript of this book was carried in my pocket over 9,000 miles, which I traveled for the purpose of securing the material and photographs contained within these pages.

I have personally met and felt the muscles of nearly all the athletes whose pictures appear in this book. I have endeavored to secure photographs of men who have spent years in the world of athletics and whose physiques show the remarkable results of their different professions. I have done this solely to arouse the reader's enthusiasm.

Because of thousands of requests which I have received from all parts of the world, this book came into being. It has been written with an unprejudiced mind and I have endeavored to tell the exact truth on muscle building, gained from years of careful observation and research, coupled with experience not only on my own body, but also on the physiques of thousands upon thousands of my pupils.

Physiology has been completely left out. I have used as few anatomical terms as possible, and these only where it is necessary. I have endeavored to explain muscle building in a simplified manner so that it could be easily understood by readers in all stages of life.

If one—just one—under-developed reader obtains a strong, robust body through following the suggestions I have outlined in this book, I will feel amply repaid for my efforts.

INTRODUCTION

THERE'S probably a time in everyone's life when he wishes he were stronger, and had more skill and endurance. This may first make itself known in boyhood, in an argument with the school bully, or it may not come until middle age, when a man realizes he is slipping backward. If you ask one hundred boys if they would like to double their present strength, you would probably receive one hundred answers in the affirmative, for the answer is revealed in the Bible adage, "The glory of young men is their strength."

If you propounded the same question to a group of men between the ages of twenty-five and thirty-five, you probably would not receive more than 50 per cent, or 60 per cent, affirmative replies, for the remainder would hesitate, or perhaps would not know. Ask the same question of one hundred men between the age of forty and fifty and the ones who are enthusiastic about increasing their strength are in the minority, for a man at this age is usually more desirous of increasing his vitality and preparing to lengthen his stay upon this earth.

Regardless of age, however, there are very few people who would refuse to increase their strength, improve their appearance, and experience all the joys of living a physical culture life, if they could acquire these things without too much effort. The plain truth of it is that most people are lazy. They will not exert a sufficient amount of energy to the care and welfare of their bodies, which, if left undone, will positively cause them to slip backward rather than go forward.

If more people realized the importance of devoting even ten to fifteen minutes daily to the care and welfare of their bodies, there would be far less dyspepsia, rheumatism, under-nourishment or obesity. If people only realized what it means to possess robust health, abounding strength and the feeling of satisfaction that accompanies a well-muscled body, physical culturists would be in the majority instead of in the minority.

I have often watched crowds pass on the streets and noticed most of the individuals shuffle along more dead than alive. Seventy-five per cent, of them are round-shouldered and flat-chested; many are carrying twenty- five to fifty pounds extra weight around their waists and hips. Once in a while you will see someone in the passing throng with a springy step, deep, full chest and straight, broad shoulders. You can tell at once that he is a physical culturist who has devoted some time to the care and welfare of his body. Your attention is attracted to him because of his personality, which is emphasized by his athletic appearance. His complexion is clear, his eyes sparkle, he radiates vitality. Lines of dissipation are absent.

Wouldn't it be wonderful if everyone looked and felt like this? Medical doctors would soon become rare and drug stores would sell fewer drugs, and even less toilet articles than they now sell. There is really no excuse for anyone who fails to enjoy all the thrills resulting from robust health. Anyone who is too lazy to devote a little time to his physical welfare deserves absolutely no sympathy when sickness or disease gets him.

It is my pleasure and great privilege to tell you in this series of little informal talks just how you can enjoy the delights of robust health and the feeling of security and satisfaction that comes to a man who knows that he can give a good account of himself in any emergency that may arise, and who has the courage and the red-blooded love of life to want to increase not only his own happiness, but also the happiness and the comfort of those who love and respect him and wish him well.

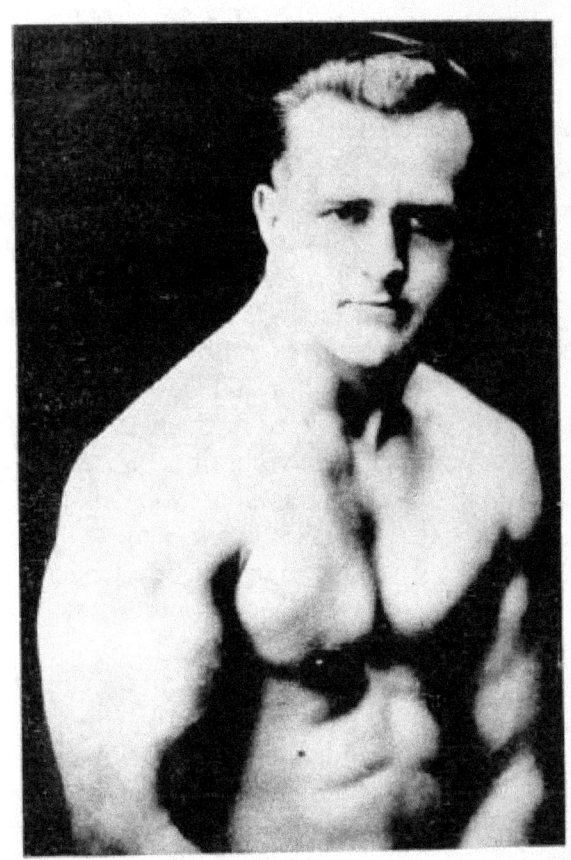

EARLE E. LIEDERMAN
Showing the physical development of the author.

Chapter I
The Various Forms of Exercise

There are many and varied forms of exercise. Nearly anyone who is experienced in physical training has his own method of performing exercises. It is difficult to suggest a course of training for anyone where the exercises would please the individual in every respect. When training, the physical culturist must take the bitter with the sweet. He must perform exercises that are not at all to his liking, and often he will find that such exercises are really the ones his muscles require the most for full development. When an exercise seems disagreeable or difficult, it is proof in itself that the muscles affected have been neglected. If you wish to perform only the exercises to your liking, you will naturally pick out the easiest work, and neglect the ones most necessary. There is frequently a tendency to fool yourself. I can relate an instance from my own experience which demonstrates this.

Years ago, when I first started active training, I outlined a course for myself. I selected what I thought to be the best possible exercises, in order to develop and strengthen my muscles. I religiously followed this system, and as I found the work becoming easier and easier, I naturally thought I was increasing rapidly in strength. However, the truth of the matter was that I was gradually discovering easier and easier methods of performing the movements, thereby not only fooling myself, but also cheating my muscles as well.

Great care should be taken, therefore, in regard to the selection of exercises, for if the student discovers easier methods of performing them, he is not only fooling himself, but he is also retarding his progress.

Don't Hypnotize Yourself with a Wrong Idea

I have often observed different individuals exercising in gymnasiums, and wondered while watching them perform light free-hand movements what physical goal they had set for themselves. I have seen some chaps swinging and twisting their arms madly, probably thinking in their minds that they were securing muscular development and strength. I have wondered how anyone could hypnotize himself in this way. Light calisthenic work has never developed huge muscles, and never will. In fact, anyone who wants to obtain the best results in the minimum of time, should bear in mind that the muscles must be exercised in groups, as well as individually. It is all very well to adopt a system of light dumb-bell exercises, but you will find that in time the work will become exceedingly monotonous.

My main objection to light dumb-bell work is that in the beginning you need only practice an exercise from ten to twenty times in order to tire the muscles, while after several months, in order to tire these muscles to the same degree, the repetitions must be continued many hundreds of counts. When you consider the time involved in exercising in this manner, the folly of it can readily be seen.

Then, again, endless repetition of movements has a tendency to wear the tissues away faster than they can be replenished. Therefore, instead of increasing the size of the muscles, they will slowly decrease, until the student possesses a body consisting of bones and long, stringy-looking muscles, not only unpleasing to the eye, but useless from the standpoint of strength. The muscles may have endurance, it is true, but that kind of endurance for only one muscle at a time is absolutely useless for the hard worker. How can anyone expect to possess co-ordination in active work when his muscles have never worked together in groups? Of what use is a biceps, for example, that can perform five hundred or one thousand flexions with a five-pound dumb-bell when put to a test, if it must seek the help of the shoulders, chest and leg muscles in some form of competition ?

What Twenty Years of Close Observation Have Taught Me

It is not my intention to condemn any system of physical culture of the present day, for every teacher has a right to his own opinion, especially when he is in earnest. However, the pointers and advice I am endeavoring to set forth in these pages are based not only upon more than twenty years of close observation and study, but also upon more than twenty years of personal experience on my own body, which is the very best experience of all. Advice should be taken from one who can show results on his own person, and everyone knows that you can learn a great deal more from a practical man than you can from a theoretical one. If a penniless tramp tried to tell you how to become a financial success, you would not heed him one-tenth as much as you would a wealthy business man. The very same thing applies to physical training. Men who really do things are the men to learn from. If the student will bear this in mind in his endeavor to seek strength and development, more rapid progress will be made.

It is not necessary for anyone to attend a gymnasium in order to perfect his body. Of course, a gymnasium is a great help, owing to the atmosphere of the place and the competition one is bound to encounter. But if one has the will power and the determination to succeed, he can accomplish even better results in the privacy of his own room, where the fullest concentration can be effected.

I am a firm believer in paying strict attention to each. Showing what a young man can do for himself if he desires extension and contraction of the muscles, for if the mind wanders, there is a tendency to slacken the effort.

In order to succeed in exercising, the student must perform progressive work. He must work a little harder each week or month in order to develop his body to its

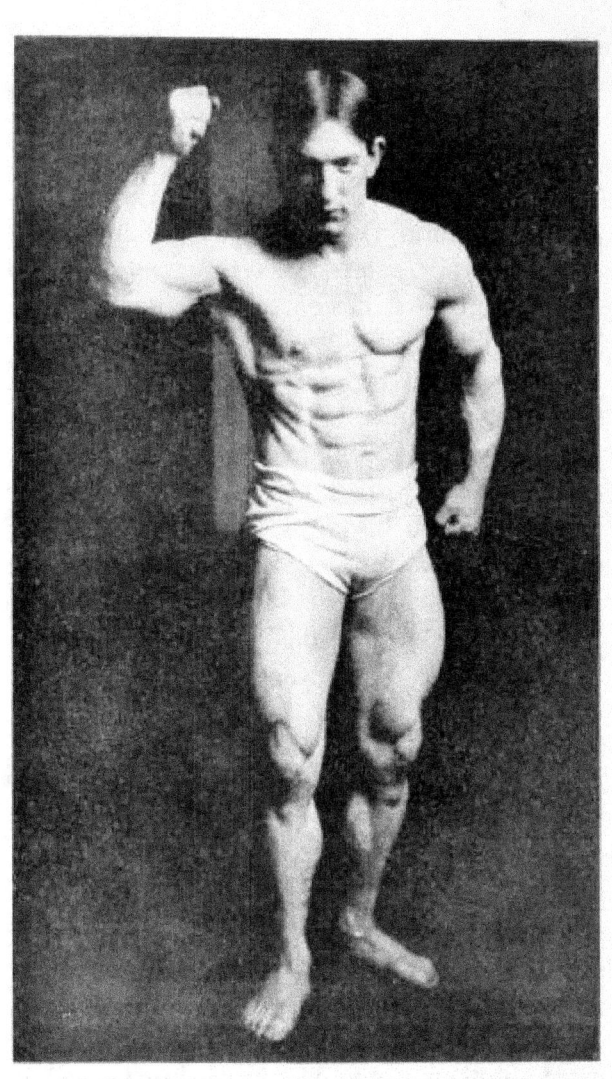

Showing what a young man can do for himself if he desires.

maximum proportions. If he does not do this, he will merely reach a certain point in development and then stand still.

The Wrong and the Right Way to Train

I remember some years ago a young man came to me asking my advice regarding the treatment of his own body. He had a fairly good physique. As I remember, his arm measured about 14 inches when flexed. This young man told me that he had been exercising a little more than three years. However, during the last year or more, he had not made any noticeable gain. Therefore, he was not only anxious, but somewhat discouraged over his progress, as naturally he would be.

I asked him what form of training he had been following, and he told me. He never gave progressive exercising a thought, but continued working every day at a monotonous drill that gave him a fairly good development, but no weight behind his muscles. He looked drawn and slim, and although he could move every muscle of his body at will, yet they were not of the kind that are pleasing to the eye. I took this man in hand and outlined a course of progressive work for him to follow, and in less than seven months his arm had increased to over 15½ inches, thereby gaining as much in that short period of time as he had gained in more than twice that time while following non-progressive methods. Today he is one of the finest built athletes in this country.

A short while ago another young chap, a student of Columbia University, came in to see me. He had done a lot of work on the rings, the parallel bars and on the horse, but had never developed any really good looking muscle. He was very much dissatisfied with his progress, notwithstanding the fact that his gym instructor had assured him that he had developed about as far as he could go.

I told him frankly that he could keep up this kind of work until feathers grew on frogs, but it wouldn't get him anywhere.

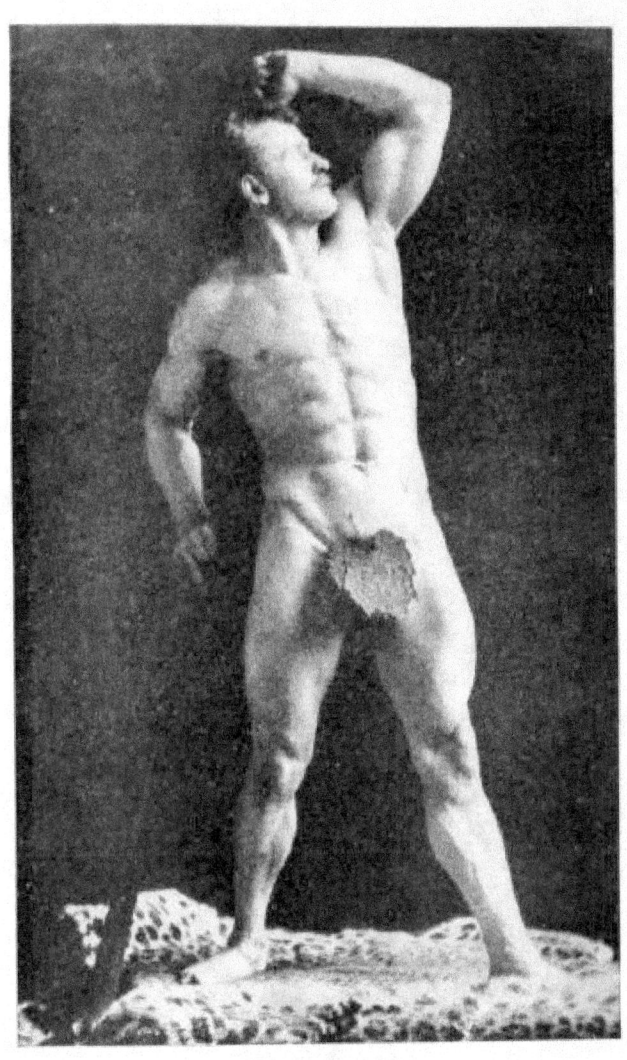

EUGEN SANDOW

The famous strong man of the past generation who without a doubt possessed a development that was as near perfection as any human being could attain. There was not a single weak spot in his make-up.

Well, to make a long story short, this chap put himself under my instruction. I gave him a carefully selected number of exercises, planned to develop his arms, chest, abdomen and legs, which he followed faithfully for three months.

At the end of this time he had gained a full inch and a half around the biceps, two inches in chest expansion and more than one inch around his thighs. Needless to say, he was delighted. I have since instructed at least a half dozen men from this man's fraternity, all of whom were equally well pleased with the results of their work.

What I Mean by Progressive Work

By progressive work I do not mean increasing the number of motions. I mean that the resistance you are working against must be made heavier as your muscles increase in strength. I am a firm believer in performing exercises that tire the muscles within ten repetitions. Of course, there are certain parts of the body that are exceptions in this case, such as the neck and thighs, possibly the abdominal region. For if too great a strain is placed upon these parts, serious results may develop. However, for the arms, chest and shoulders the student should never perform any movement that requires more than ten repetitions in order to tire the muscles if rapid gain in development is the object. The neck should be tired in less than twenty-five repetitions, likewise the thighs and the abdominal muscles.

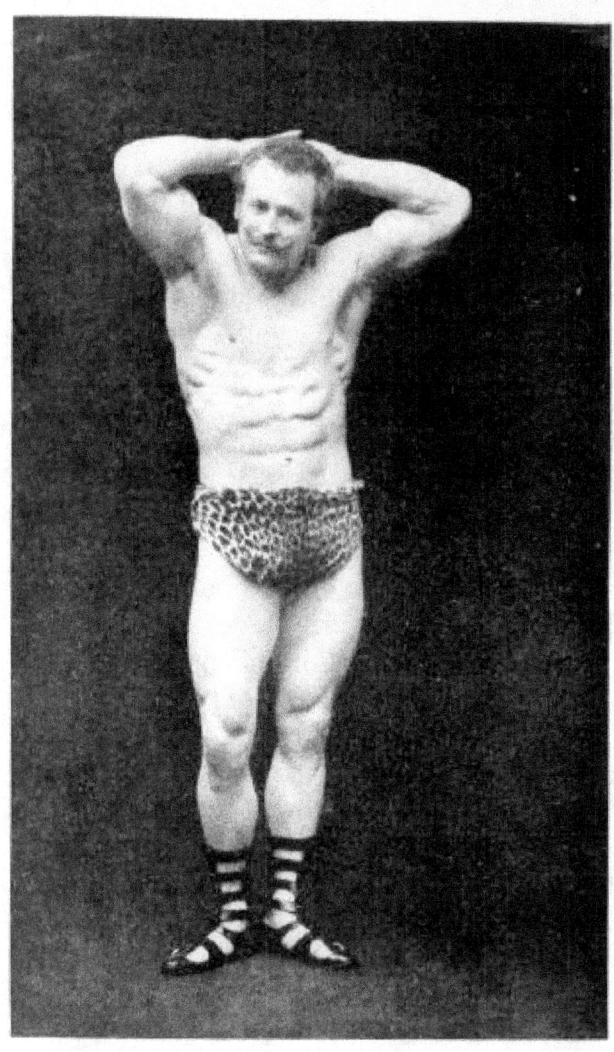

EUGEN SANDOW

The finishing touch to Sandow's perfect development was his wonderful thick arms which set off his well balanced figure.

Concentrate Your Mind on Your Work

The average beginner is ignorant regarding the proper method of performing his exercise. Just as there is a right and a wrong way to lift weights, swim, skate or perform any feat of strength or skill, so there is a right and a wrong way to exercise. In exercising, the muscles should be worked in a natural manner. For example, when exercising your biceps, the concentration and the effort should be placed on the contraction and not on the extension. To make this clearer: if you are holding a weight in your hand with your arm hanging by your side, when you bend your arm, bend it with vigor and force, concentrating upon what you are doing, until your biceps is flexed and the arm is completely bent. Do not concentrate your effort on any resistance when relaxing the arm again and lowering the weight to arm's length at your side.

Another example: When you are chinning the bar, start by hanging on the bar with your arms straight. Then endeavor to bring your chin over the bar by flexing the arms and pulling the body upwards. Concentration and vigor should be put on this upward pull, while you should lower yourself in a natural, relaxed way. I have seen athletes perform the exercise of chinning the bar and have noticed how slowly they have lowered themselves, seeming to pay special attention to the flexed state of their arms while lowering the body. If they paid more attention to pulling their bodies upwards, much better results could be accomplished. Try this for yourself the next time you happen to be in the gym, and see what a difference it will make.

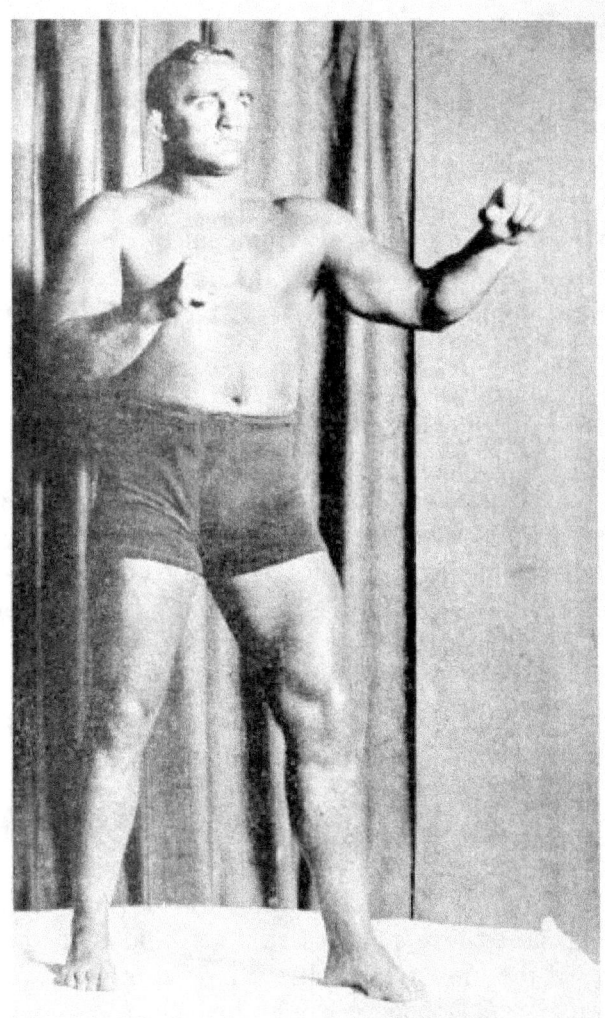

WLADEK ZBYSZKO

This remarkable wrestler not only has splendid proportions, but his muscles are capable of prolonged endurance. He can handle his weight, 220 pounds, with the ease of a lightweight. Smooth type, yet possessing bulky muscles.

The triceps muscle, back of the arms, works just the reverse of the biceps. Therefore, when you push any object overhead, concentrate and use force in the movement. Pay no particular attention to the lowering of the weight to the shoulder again. In other words, use the muscles in their own natural way, the way in which they were intended to be used. The biceps muscle was meant to flex the arm and the triceps muscle to extend the arm. The same thing applies to any muscle of the body. Later on I will go into this matter more completely.

The Size of the Bones Makes a Big Difference

The size of the bones is an important factor in determining the contour and shape, as well as the size of the muscles. That is why a person who has a small framework can hardly expect to equal the proportions of a large-boned individual, although I have seen phenomenally developed athletes with small bones.

Nevertheless, it is a fact that a large-boned man can become much stronger and have much larger muscles than his small-boned competitor. The small-boned man, however, has the advantage over a large-boned individual in the fact that he can develop muscles that are much more pleasing to the eye, and which will make him look much larger in photographs than anyone who has a large frame. This is because of his small wrist, elbow and knee joints.

One of the most remarkable examples I have ever seen of this was in a young man who had but a 6¾-inch wrist and whose upper arm measured a trifle over 16 inches when flexed. His chest and back and legs also reached enormous proportions. This chap was but 5 feet 6 inches in height and weighed in the neighborhood of 165 pounds. If, with all the work he had done to obtain this phenomenal development, he had had large bones, he would have undoubtedly become one of the world's strongest and most muscular men. In photographs, however, he looked much

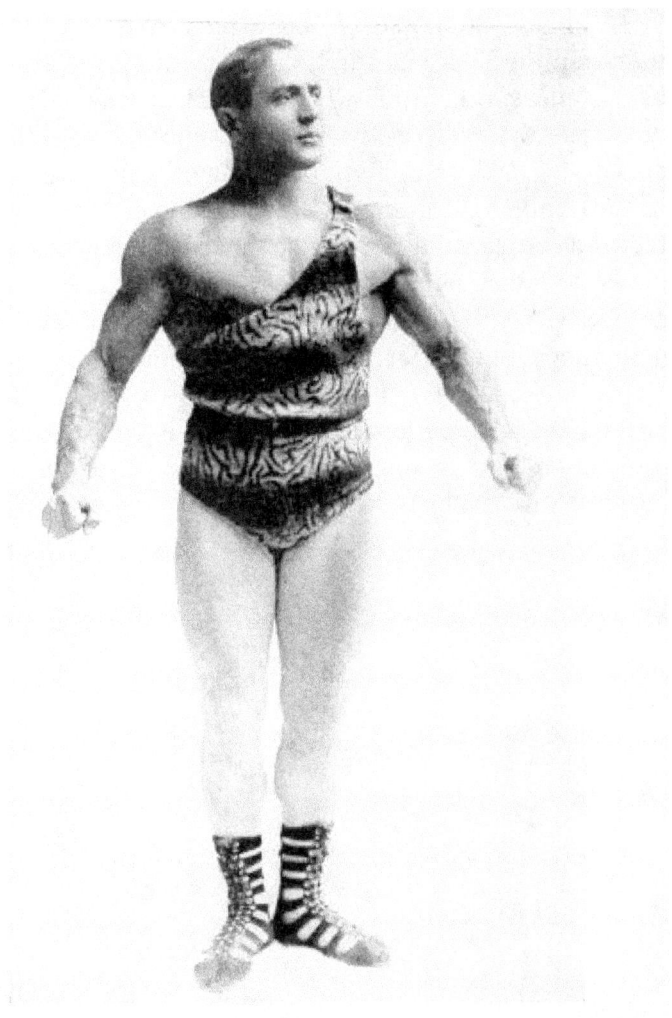

ABE BOSHES

A highly developed strong man whose muscles are well proportioned and supple. He is an example proving that a small-boned man can easily attain herculean proportions by proper exercise. An interesting study of the deltoid muscles can be had from this photograph. When the deltoids are highly developed they add several inches to the breadth of the shoulders.

better developed and much stronger than some of the world's record holders, who nearly always have been men of large bones.

A man who possesses an 8-inch wrist and who will train faithfully for several years, will eventually have a biceps measuring from 17 to 18 inches when flexed, and other parts of his body in the same huge proportions, providing, of course, he is of average height. Anyone who has a small, light frame should be consoled greatly by the fact that he can develop much finer looking muscles than his large-boned neighbor. His muscles will stand out better and he will have better control of them. He will also make a better appearance than his big, husky competitor.

So cheer up, if you happen to be of slight frame, for faithful, regular performance of your exercises may bring rewards to you in muscular appearance that you couldn't get if you were a heavyweight.

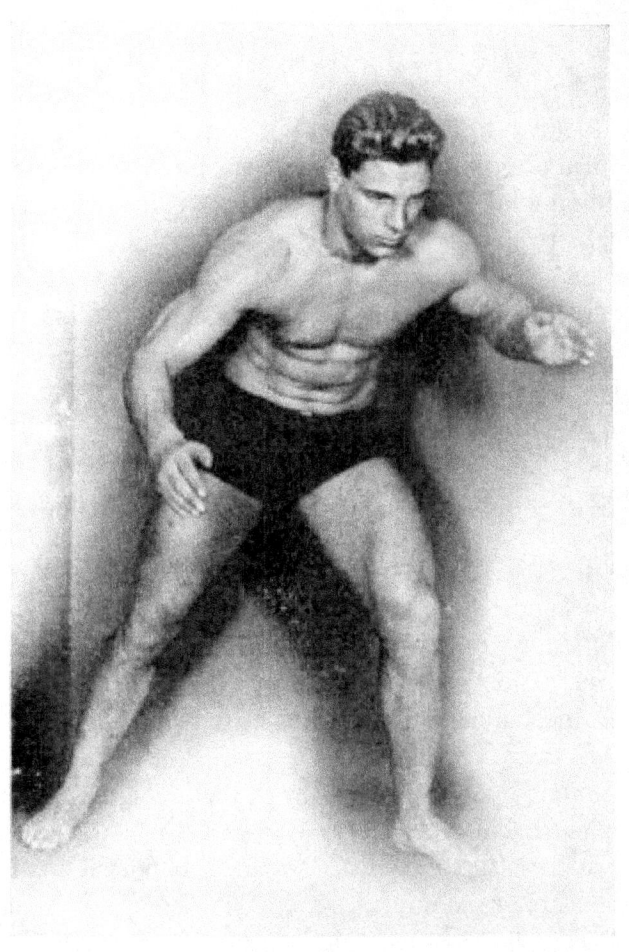

G. CALZA

A strong young wrestler whose muscles are panther-like in quickness. The author has watched the work of this mat artist and has marveled at the wonderful endurance and strength he has shown in his contests.

Chapter II
The Ideal Measurements

I WAS down in Florida one winter at a time when quite a bunch of motion picture stars and professional people were vacationing at the winter playground. A little crowd of us were gathered on the beach doing various athletic stunts—and believe me, some of those chaps were mighty clever.

After we got tired of our sport, we sat around on the sand talking, and finally the subject came up as to what should be the ideal measurements for a man.

One of the party spoke up and said: "This is a subject that is hard to agree upon. The proportions of the old Greek sculptors for men varied a great deal. For instance, take the Farnese Hercules, the Apollo Belvedere, the Laocoon group—there's such a wide margin of variation that you have to accept measurements based on some given type.

"While all women can aspire, at some given age, to the Venus de Milo, or the Juno type, to classify a man for accurate measurements you have to picture him as one of three or four very distinct types. And naturally, his measurements will correspond with the ideal measurements of some particular type."

I then spoke up and said: "My ideal is not the man with the huge, abnormal muscles of a Hercules; nor is it the lithe, slender form of an Apollo; nor the somewhat better-muscled Mercury. I like to see big, firm muscles, combined with speed and flexibility. The question goes even deeper than this. When holding up an ideal for scores of thousands to copy after, we set the following requisites:

"A man should look good from every angle. He should have curves and contour rather than great, disfiguring ridges of muscle. He should have a development which is possible for attainment by almost any average boy or young man, who will apply himself to development and cultivate strength, speed and perfect health."

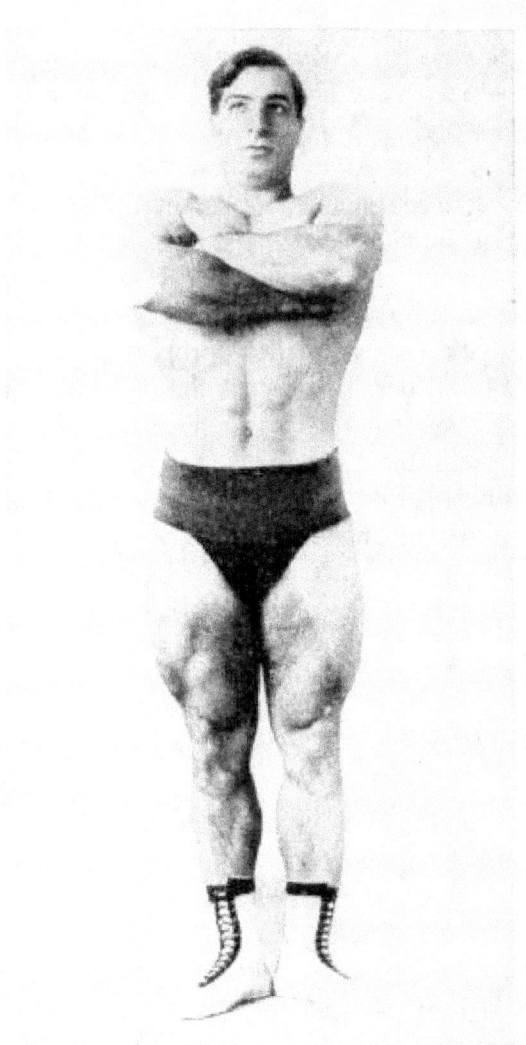

WILLIAM GERARDI

This plate was made from a print, yet it displays the largest thigh development ever seen by the author. Mr. Gerardi's thigh measures over 31 inches. He is remarkably strong, and despite his enormous bulk, is quick in his movements.

This made quite an impression on the crowd, and suggested to me the title of this chapter.

The Ideal to Which You Should Aspire

Now, I want to say right here that it is exceedingly difficult to set any standard of measurements which the student can use as a guide for comparison in order to determine to what extent he should develop his muscles. When you take into consideration the different sizes of the bones of different individuals, and combine this with hereditary conditions, it is, in my opinion, practically impossible to set any standard of measurements. You can, however, work out a standard of proportion where each part of the body will bear its proper relation to the others. Even though the student should not obtain these relative proportions, still there is no reason why he cannot possess a beautiful physique by approaching the following, which is my idea of how a man should be proportionately built:

Average height	5 feet 8 inches to 5 feet 9 inches
Neck	17 inches
Biceps	16 inches
Calf	15 inches
Chest normal	44 inches
Waist	32 inches
Thigh	23½ inches

My reason for mentioning the neck, upper arm and calves first is that the common conception of Grecian proportions stipulates the neck, upper arm flexed, and calf to be of the same size, with which I do not agree. If an individual possessed a 17-inch neck, and a 17-inch arm, he would undoubtedly possess a phenomenal development. But if he also had a 17-inch calf, it would spoil his proportions, as it would make him look much too heavy in the legs.

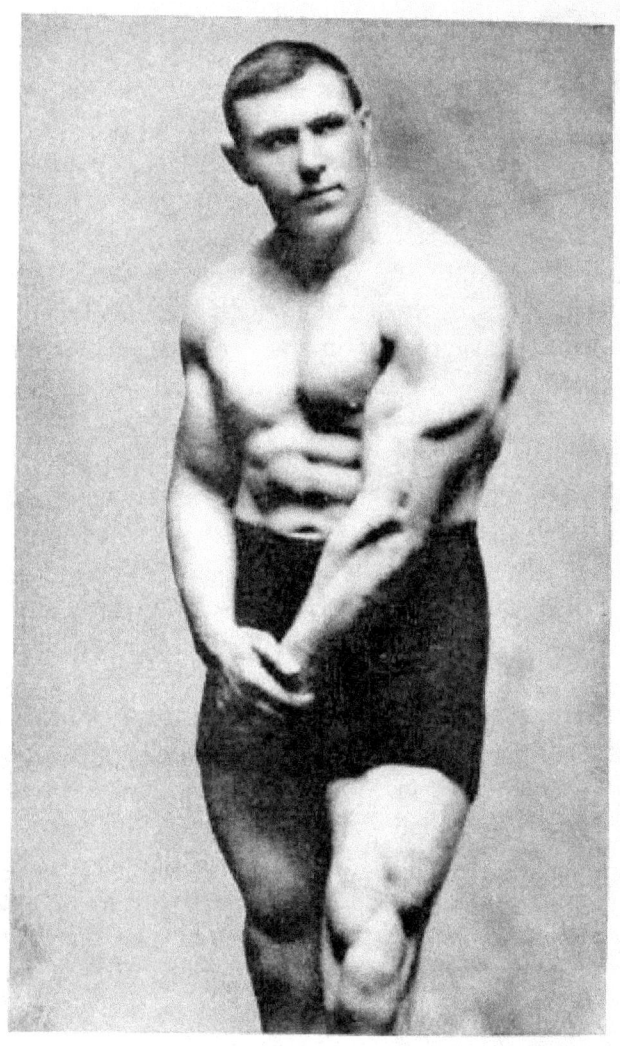

I have found by observation and careful study that the athletes who taper down slightly are more pleasing to look upon than those whose legs are of huge dimensions, like the Farnese Hercules, for instance. Therefore, in order to taper down, the neck should be a little larger than the arm, and the arm a little larger than the calf.

Now, if a person has a 16-inch neck, his arm should measure 15 inches, and his calf about 14 inches. If the individual has any smaller measurements than these, taking for granted that he is of average height, he would be too slim a type to attract attention in the physical culture world, as far as strength and development are concerned. A man with an 18-inch neck, and 17-inch arm, and a 16-inch calf would be very gigantic in size, and undoubtedly he would be exceptionally strong.

You very seldom see 17-inch arms and 18-inch necks on persons of average height, for athletes possessing these enormous measurements usually are in the neighborhood of 6 feet tall. There are, of course, many exceptions to this, especially among wrestlers.

For instance, George Hackenschmidt had an enormous neck. I have seen measurements for this part of his body and these measurements are given by different authorities all the way from 19½ inches to 22 inches. Unfortunately I have not had the pleasure of measuring Mr. Hackenschmidt, consequently I do not care to express my opinion of the actual size of his neck. However, I did have the pleasure of feeling his arm, and although my own hands are of medium size, still I could not span the breadth of his upper arm when I felt it. I have seen measurements of his upper arm given by different authorities as being anywhere from 18 inches to 19¾ inches. The reader will, therefore, note that no matter how Hackenschmidt's measurements may vary in accordance with different writers, still everyone mentioned the difference in size between the neck and the upper arms.

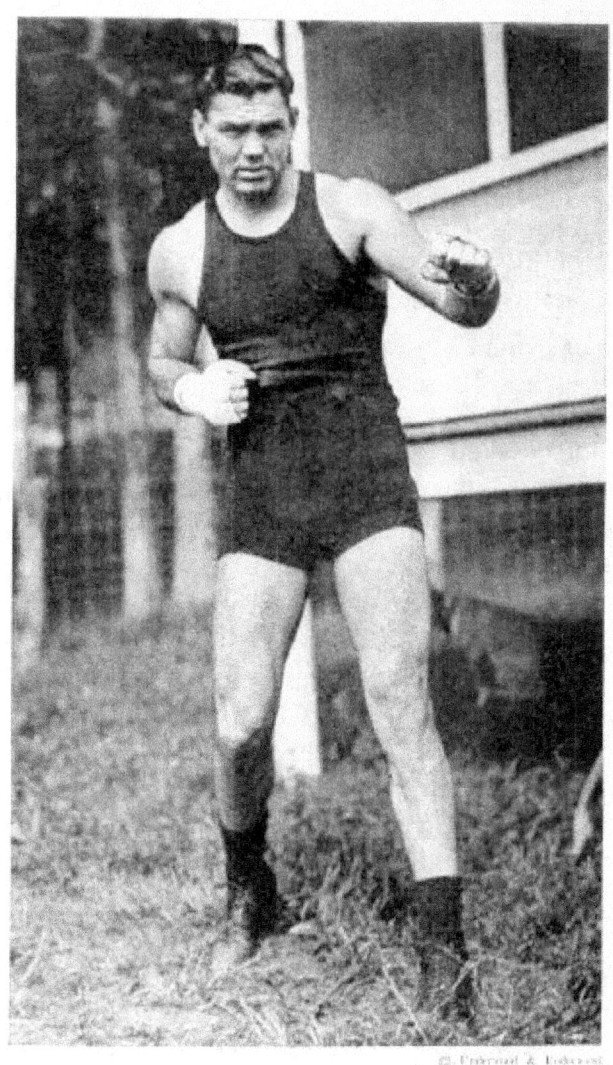

JACK DEMPSEY

The former champion was the greatest fighting machine the world has ever produced. He is symmetrically proportioned and the wonderful co-ordination of his muscles can only be told by his long record of knockouts.

Hackenschmidt was a rare exception in muscular development and strength, and I want to make it clear that no matter how diligently a person may work, there is not one athlete in ten thousand who could ever acquire Hackenschmidt's proportions and strength.

The Size of the Head Is an Important Factor

The size of the head is an important factor covering neck measurements. Therefore, if the individual has a long, narrow head, and is of a slender type, it will be a physical impossibility for him ever to attain a neck much over 17 inches, providing, of course, he is of average height. By average height, I mean people ranging from 5 feet 7 to 5 feet 9 inches. If the individual is near 6 feet, or even over, naturally he will have larger measurements than the individual of only average height. However, if he is below the average in height, say 5 feet 3 or 4 inches, he must not expect to attain the measurements of an individual of 5 feet 9 inches in height. In other words, the taller you are, the larger your measurements should be, providing, of course, that you adopt scientific progressive training and work faithfully to reach your goal.

Although I mentioned 44 inches normal chest measurement, yet it is exceedingly difficult to standardize any chest measurement to correspond with a 17-inch neck, for, owing to the different formation of everyone's torso, the measurement of the chest varies as much as 4 inches in the normal girth. Greater variation will be found in the expanded chest measurement. All I can say on the subject is that anyone with a 17-inch neck and 16- inch upper arm when flexed, should have a chest normal of over 43 inches.

The waist also varies in size according to the frame and width of the hips, and also the muscular development of the individual. A student who has devoted considerable attention to his waist muscles, especially those at the sides of his waist and lower back, naturally will have at least an inch larger waist than a person who has neglected this part of his body, taking for granted, of course, that the waist is free of all superfluous flesh.

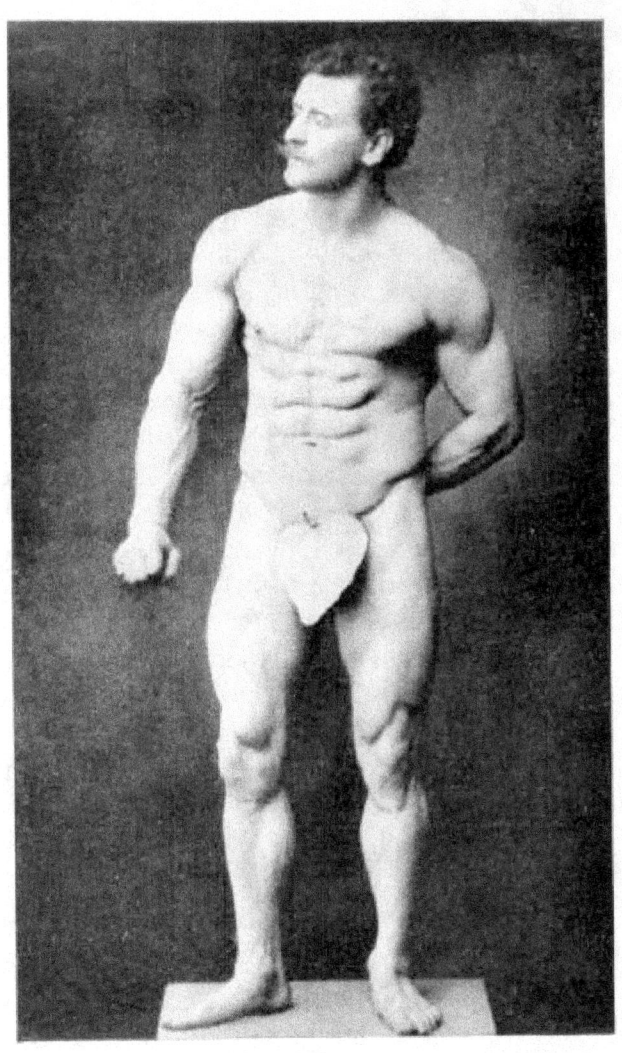

EUGEN SANDOW
A study of this famous strong man taken when he toured this country in 1893

Again, the height of the individual is an important factor in the size of the waist measurement. A 6-foot man with a waist measuring less than 33 inches would, in my opinion, appear weak, while a man of average height, whose waist measured less than 31 inches, would also appear weak. On the other hand, if the individual was but 5 feet 3 or 4 inches in height, and if he possessed a waist of 27 or 28 inches, he would still be in splendid proportions.

I Failed to Reach My Earlier Ideal

I have often thought how discouraged a student must be who has exercised faithfully month after month, and even for several years, and failed to reach the measurements he had set in mind as his goal. I can only tell you the story of my own experience, which undoubtedly corresponds with thousands of others under similar circumstances. When I first became interested in physical education, I studied photographs and the measurements of all professional strong men whose data I could secure. I noted the enormous chest measurements given by some of these prominent strong men, many of them reaching almost 60 inches around the chest when expanded. I envied those whose normal chests measured anywhere from 47 to over 50 inches. I longed to possess a chest like theirs.

I have worked faithfully for many years; yet I fall far short of these measurements. Today my normal chest measurement is but 44¾ inches, and my chest measurement, expanded, reaches 48¾ inches. Many times during my period of body-building I became discouraged because my measurements were so slow in reaching the goal I had set for them.

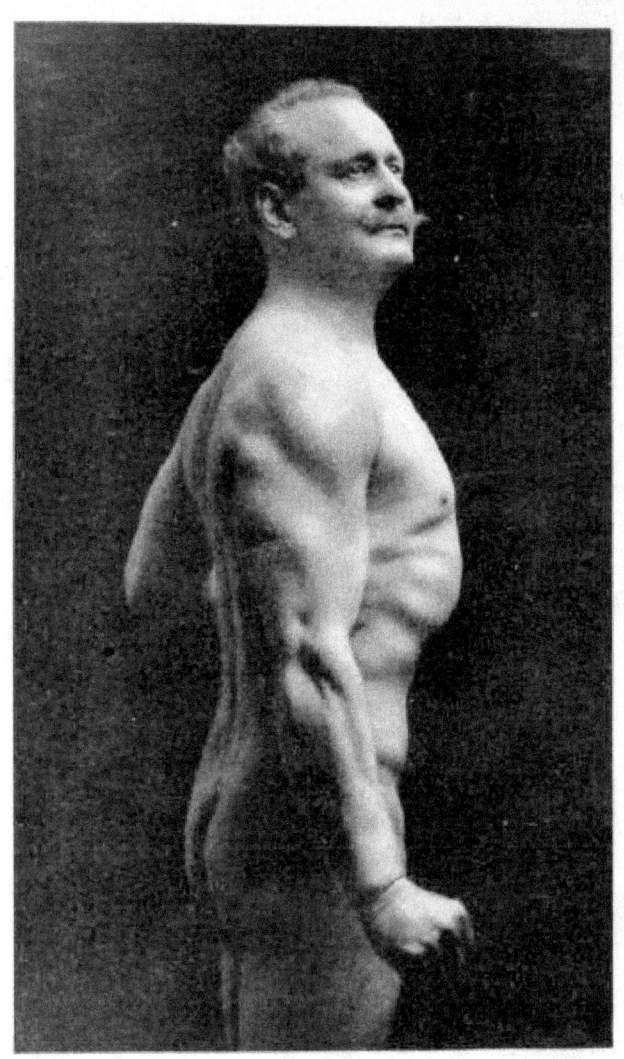

EUGEN SANDOW

When I shook hands and said goodby to Mr. Sandow in London, just before his sudden accidental death, I told him my ambition was to look as he did when I became 58 years old. I don't think there is one single reader whose ambitions are not the same as mine.— E. L.

I was also always anxious to obtain flexed biceps measuring 17¾ inches or 18 inches, but again I fell short of these proportions. Today my flexed upper arm measures but 16¾ inches. If the reader should experience any similar discouragement, let me console him with the fact that 90 per cent, of the measurements given out by famous professional strong men are grossly exaggerated. I know personally several athletes prominent in the physical culture world who claim 49-inch normal chests and 17-inch upper arms when, in reality, their chest normal is many inches less and their upper arms are not as large as my own.

Only a few months ago a crowd of us were gathered in the private gym of a well-known boxing trainer when this shy subject came up. The boxing instructor, one of the finest developed men of his class, and one of prominence as well, was telling about some of the famous athletes of a former generation, when he happened to mention Matsada Sarakichi.

Some of my middle-aged readers may recall this Sarakichi, a Japanese wrestler of phenomenal development, with the strength of an ox. The boxing master had a framed photo of this athlete hanging on the wall, near his desk. Pointing to the picture, he said: "How much would you boys say Matsada measured around the chest?"

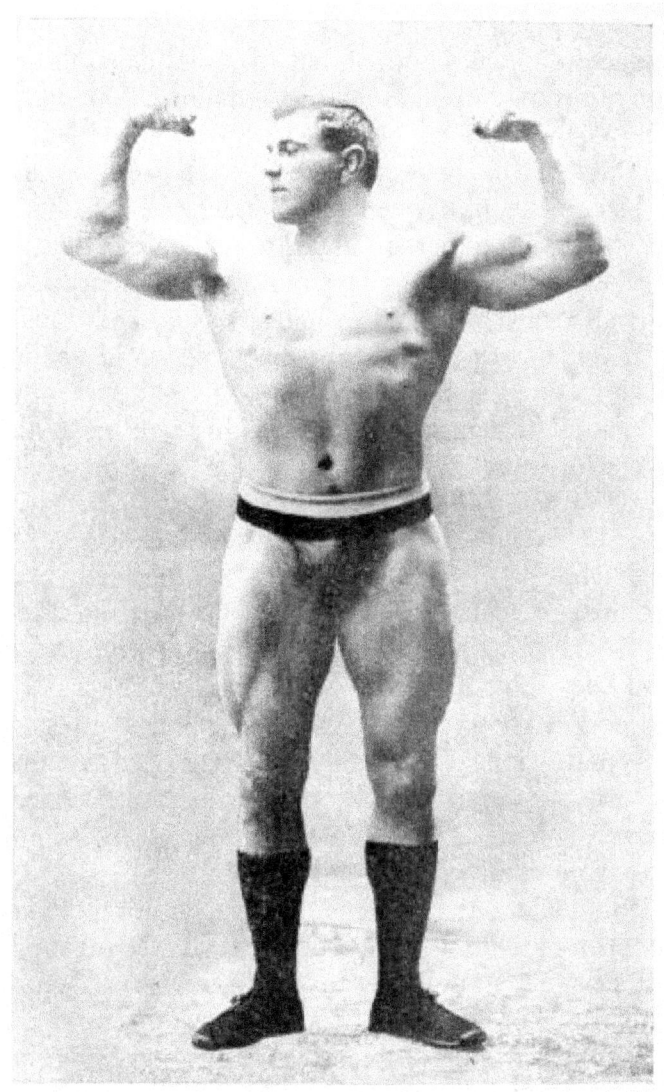

The Jap was about 5 feet 11 inches in height and he looked as though he weighed just about a pound less than a horse; so we guessed him—50 to 54 inches.

"You're all wrong," said the old boxer. "He only measured 47 inches normal, but when he folded those great arms of his over his chest and puffed himself out, he looked as big as a whale."

And that's the answer. It isn't the size, so much as what the size looks like when it's photographed. I shall have something very important to say to you about this subject a little later on that may give you a lot of help in presenting yourself to the public in a more pleasing and convincing form. But I want to tell you something further about this question of measurements.

First and foremost I can't find it in my heart to blame a student for becoming discouraged if he does not obtain the proportions some men claim they have. I became discouraged myself, and I know just how other conscientious men, who have been working hard on their physical development, would naturally feel about the matter.

Don't Fool Yourself in Your Measuring

I do not know whether the measurements given out by some professional strong men are magnified for the purpose of self-gratification, or whether they measured themselves and actually fooled themselves in taking their measurements.

If the latter should be the case, let me warn the student that when measuring any part of his body, he must pay the most strict attention to the tape and see that it does not sag in any part. For instance, if you are measuring your chest, it is the simplest thing to fool yourself when passing the tape around and under your armpits, and then taking a deep inhalation, to throw your shoulders back and expand your chest as much as possible. Of course you see the tape measure in front of you, but if you could see the tape behind your back, you might observe that it is displaced many inches downward towards your waist.

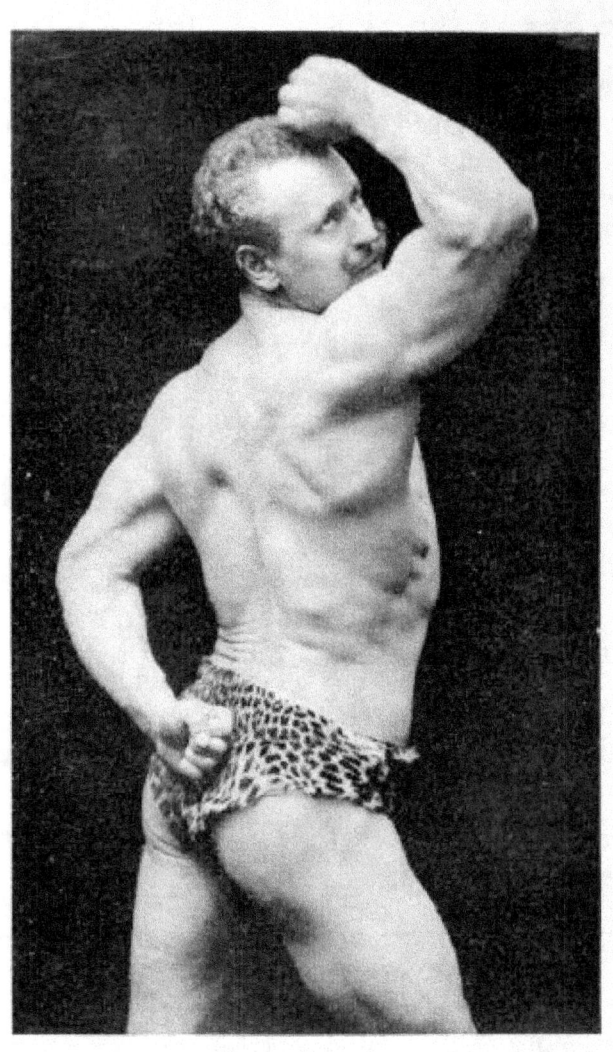

EUGEN SANDOW

This picture was taken when Sandow was about 50 years old and shows the perfect harmonious development that should put many a has-been to shame.

Always measure yourself in front of a mirror, turning around so that you can see your back as well as your front. If you have the tape fitting snugly, with about two or three pounds pressure, you will obtain your actual measurements. If these measurements fall far short of the measurements you see on paper concerning many professional strong men, do not be discouraged, for if you possess a well developed physique, you may be almost as large as these strong men are themselves.

The same thing applies to feats of strength. I do not know at the present writing how many claimants there are to the title "Strongest man in the world," but there are more claimants to this title than there are feet in a mile. As soon as an athlete obtains a little publicity and is able to lift somewhere around 250 pounds, another "world's strongest man" is found, and naturally more discouraged would-be strong men.

The Story of the Champion Lifter

It was only recently, at a weight-lifting tournament, that a well-known lifter sent in his best lifts ahead of his appearance. I chanced to see his letter and his phenomenal records actually scared me, for I had contemplated entering this tournament myself, purely for the fun of it. However, I diplomatically kept out of it as I really was afraid of this entrant. I was asked to act as a judge in this contest, as long as I did not enter it.

I expected great things from this wonderful strong man. Therefore, you can imagine my surprise when the best lift made at this open competition was only 220 pounds! In all fairness to the competitors, I am sure they could have done better, but the reader can imagine my consternation when a 220-pound lift secured a championship gold belt, when I myself had many times lifted in practice more than this. I simply mention this occurrence as it is a similar case to what I have to say on measurements.

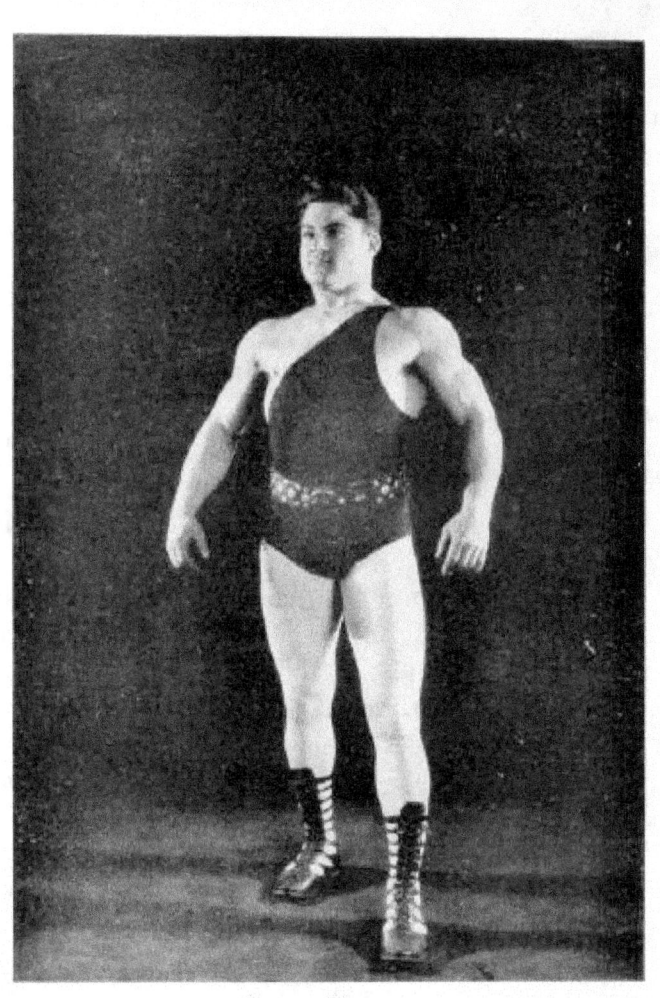

JOSEPH VITOLE

The world's record holder in the teeth lift. The remarkably strong neck this athlete possesses, combined with the bull-dog grip with his jaws, enabled him to recently lift 550 pounds with his teeth alone. When one considers Vitole's own weight being but 150 pounds, the lift is even a greater achievement.

It is a sad thing for me to tell the reader not to believe all he hears regarding feats of strength and measurements of prominent strong men. Do not misunderstand me, and think that I am including all strong men in this category.

Such men as Arthur Saxon, George Hackenschmidt, Joe Nordquest, and many others, did not exaggerate their feats of strength nor the size of their measurements—they did not have to. There are hundreds of others, too, whose records and measurements are absolutely reliable.

Let the student continue diligently with his training and endeavor to secure as well-muscled proportions as possible. Even if he does not obtain measurements any larger than my own, do not let him feel discouraged. Any young man who is from 5 feet 8 inches to 5 feet 10 inches in height should have no difficulty in obtaining at least a 16-inch upper arm and a 17-inch neck, as well as a 46 or 47-inch expanded chest. If the student is around 6 feet in height, he should have no difficulty in eventually obtaining a 17½-inch neck, a 49-inch expanded chest and a 16½-inch upper arm.

If the student is but 5 feet 3 inches or 4 inches in height, he should have no difficulty in obtaining a 16- inch neck, a 15-inch upper arm and a 44-inch expanded chest. Of the three above-mentioned groups many obtain measurements even beyond the ones I have outlined, for it is not impossible. But they should not expect to reach the Herculean proportions of a Hackenschmidt.

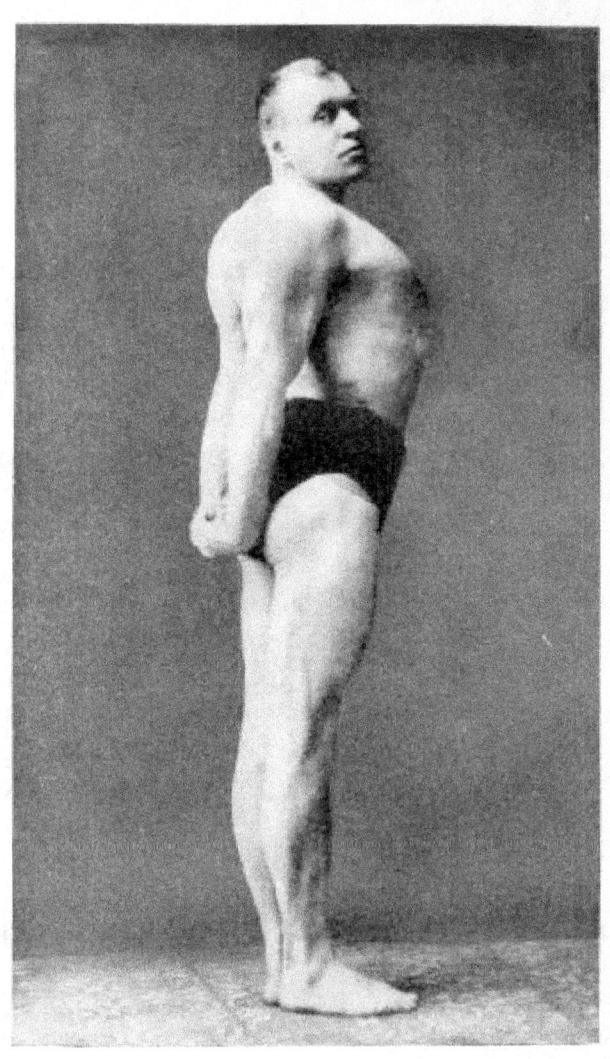

GEORGE LURICH

A strong man with a wonderful chest expansion. Besides creating records in weight-lifting, he was an accomplished wrestler and gymnast

How to Measure Your Muscles

When measuring your muscles, the tape should be passed around the largest part. Let us begin with the neck. To obtain the proper measurement of the neck, the head should be held erect, chin to the front and the tape passed around the lower part of the neck, just above the point where the trapezius muscle begins to slope towards the shoulder. Place about two pounds pressure on the tape in taking these measurements.

If you bend the head back and throw out the muscles of the neck, the neck will increase about one or two inches in size. However, you will not be obtaining your actual neck measurements, but will be obtaining a measurement of your expanded neck. You should never consider the expanded neck measurement, for in all measurement tables given of athletes, the normal neck measurement is always taken for granted. If you consider your expanded neck measurement and develop your other muscles in proportion to this, your neck will never be properly developed, for you are utilizing your expanded measurement in your table of proportions.

In measuring the chest, the tape should be passed under the armpits, in a straight line around the chest, about one inch above the nipples. By exhaling all the air from your lungs and relaxing all your muscles, you obtain your contracted chest measurement. Now adjust the tape again to the previous position and stand perfectly normal, head erect, muscles relaxed and chest corresponding with your erect standing or walking posture. This will be your normal chest girth.

By inhaling as much air as you possibly can, and at the same time expanding your latissimus dorsi muscles and swelling your chest to its utmost, you will obtain your expanded chest measurement. These measurements, of course, will not be measurements of your actual lung expansion, because they are assisted by your muscles.

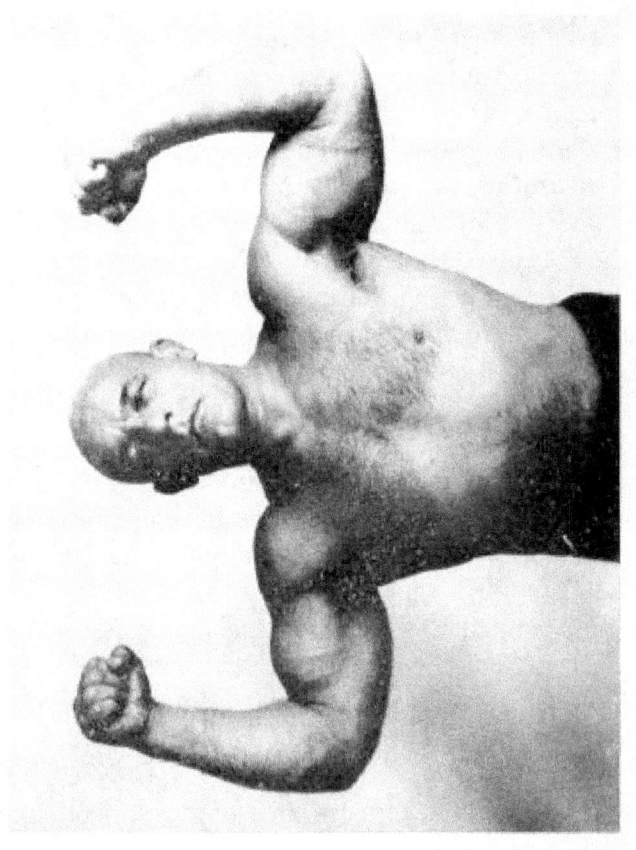

STANISLAUS ZBYSZKO

The elder brother of the famous wrestler whose gigantic proportions are almost unbelievable. Large of bone, he undoubtedly possesses the largest measurements of any trained athlete. His upper arm measures over 21 inches, while his chest is well in the fifties. When one considers his age—50 years, he is a wrestler to be marveled at.

To obtain the actual measurement of your lung expansion, you should pass the tape around your lower chest at the ninth rib, which is a few inches below the nipples. The difference between your normal and expanded chest measurements at this point will be very slight. In fact, if you expand three or more inches, you have wonderful expansion. However, these lower chest measurements are rarely utilized in any table of measurements of athletes.

How to Measure the Index of Strength

Your upper arm may rightly be regarded as your index of strength. If a chap has any development worth talking about, it usually shows in the upper arm.

In measuring your upper arm, first pass the tape around the largest part of your upper arm when the arm is straight and held relaxed horizontally. Next, flex your arm by vigorously contracting the triceps and biceps, bringing the fist as near the shoulder as possible, and turning the palm of your hand towards shoulder. By doing this, you will obtain the largest girth of your flexed upper arm, providing, of course, you pass the tape around your largest part.

In measuring your upper arm, in this case, do it before a mirror, so that you can see both the back and the front, and note whether the tape is passed straight around the arm, or whether it is on a slant. By having the tape slanting, you only fool yourself. I am convinced that it is undoubtedly just such a slanting tape that produces the magnified measurements of a great many professional strong men.

The forearms should be measured also around the largest part with the arms straight and fist clenched. To obtain the contracted forearm measurement, bend your arm and pass the tape around the largest part as near the elbow as possible.

The waist should be measured when standing in an erect posture, not drawing in too much, neither should you allow your abdomen to protrude. By holding the chest up in a military carriage, you will obtain your normal waist measurement. The tape should be passed around the waist at about the height of the navel.

In measuring the hips, pass the tape around the largest part and apply about four pounds pressure, thus allowing for irregularities of this part of the body.

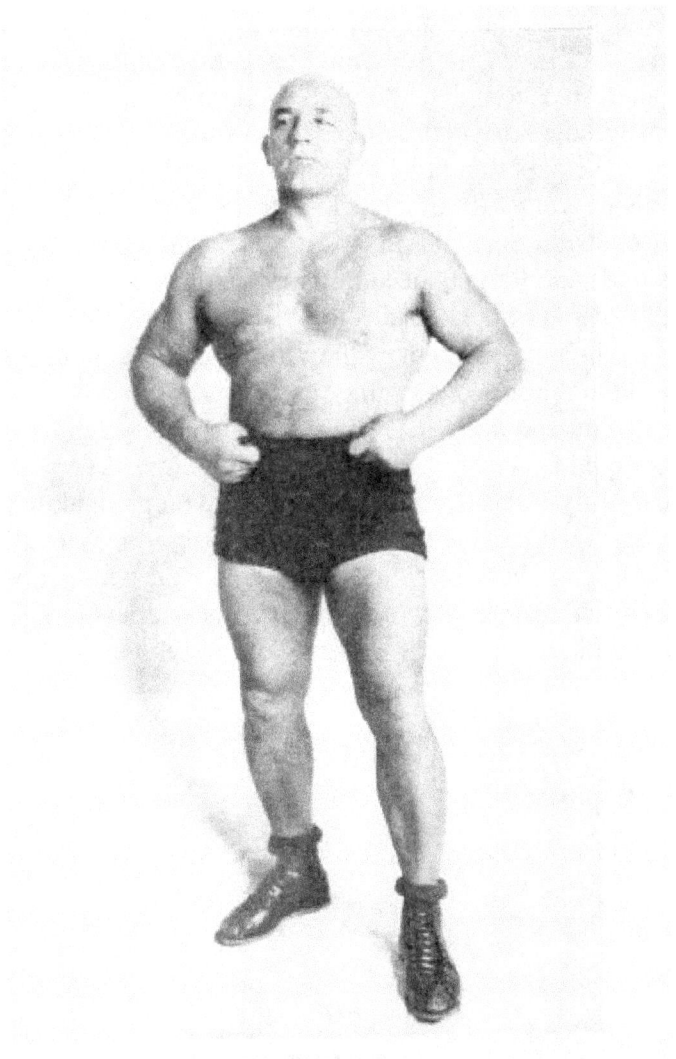

STANISLAUS ZBYSZKO

The gigantic proportions of this 245-pound man can hardly be appreciated because of his large bones and large head.

The measurement of the thighs should be taken around the largest part of the thigh, which in most cases is directly below the crotch. If your legs are exceptionally developed, with pronounced curves to the extensor muscles, perhaps your largest girth may be a little lower than this. However, this can be easily ascertained and the measurement can be taken in a complete state of contraction; that is, when you stiffen the knee and tighten the muscles.

The calf should be measured around the largest part. By raising your toes off the floor and simply standing on your heels, you will obtain a slightly larger girth than if you stood flat footed, because you can get a slightly greater expansion of the muscles in this position.

The measurement of the wrist and ankle should be taken around the smallest girth.

You should, when you begin your development, take a complete set of these measurements, keeping them carefully, so as to see what progress you are making. In this way you'll be able to get a mental picture of yourself, at any time, just the way you were before you commenced your training, and surprise all your friends with the progress you are making.

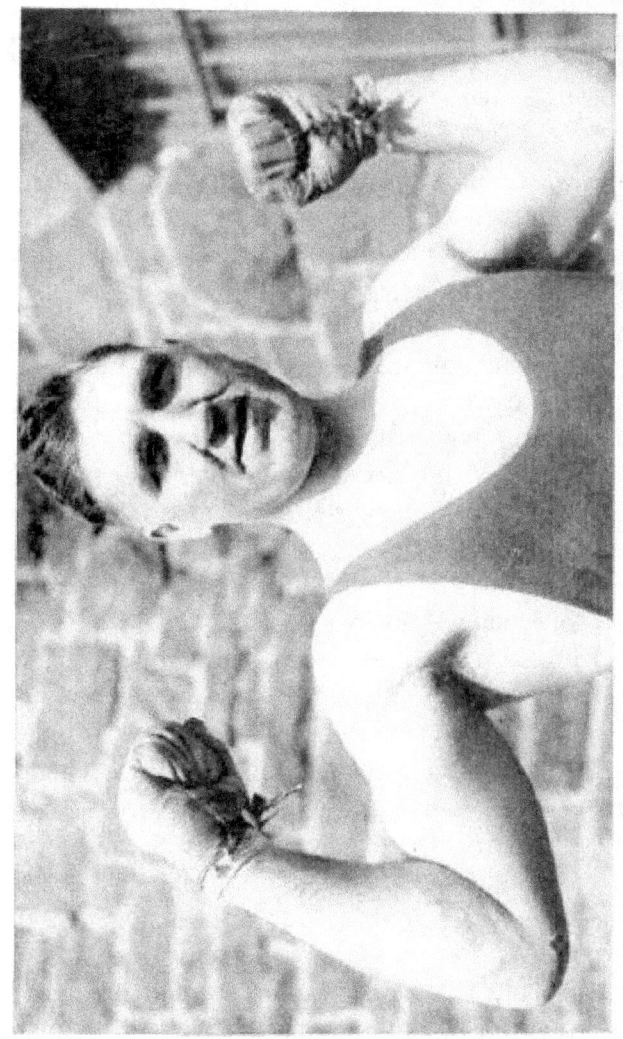

JESS WILLARD

Undoubtedly the biggest fighter who ever became champion. His 6 feet 7 inches of height naturally gives him an enormous reach, yet his arms are remarkably thick. The above pose interestingly indicates the lack of knotty muscles in a fighter's development.

© Underwood & Underwood

Chapter III
The Structure and Development of the Neck

A SHORT time ago I was talking on physical development to a well-known athlete. This man had broken into the game as a hammer-thrower and shot-putter during his college career, but subsequently wound up as one of the best mat artists in the country.

He had a magnificent development, which I admired very much, so we got to discussing the various things that go to build up a powerful physique that is "easy to look at." In the course of the conversation this man said to me: "You can talk as you please, but I as an athlete judge a man's development more by the size and contour of his neck than by any other way. For what a man is, and what he has done, shows up in his neck, and in the full, firm contour of these muscles just as though he had drawn a map for you."

What my friend said is true, for the neck is one part of the body that responds very rapidly to exercise, and a well-developed neck is not only pleasing to the eye, but helps greatly to convey a better blood supply to the brain. Then, too, it has its advantages in the event of a fall, for a strong neck is not as apt to break as a weak one. In order to develop the neck to pleasing proportions, a great variety of movements must be gone through, for much finer results can be accomplished by varying the movements than if the student simply performed one or two exercises.

Don't Try to Choke Yourself

The wearing of tight collars retards neck development. Collars should be worn comfortably, not too loose so as to look untidy. Soft collars are much better to wear than stiff starched collars, for they allow greater freedom of movement.

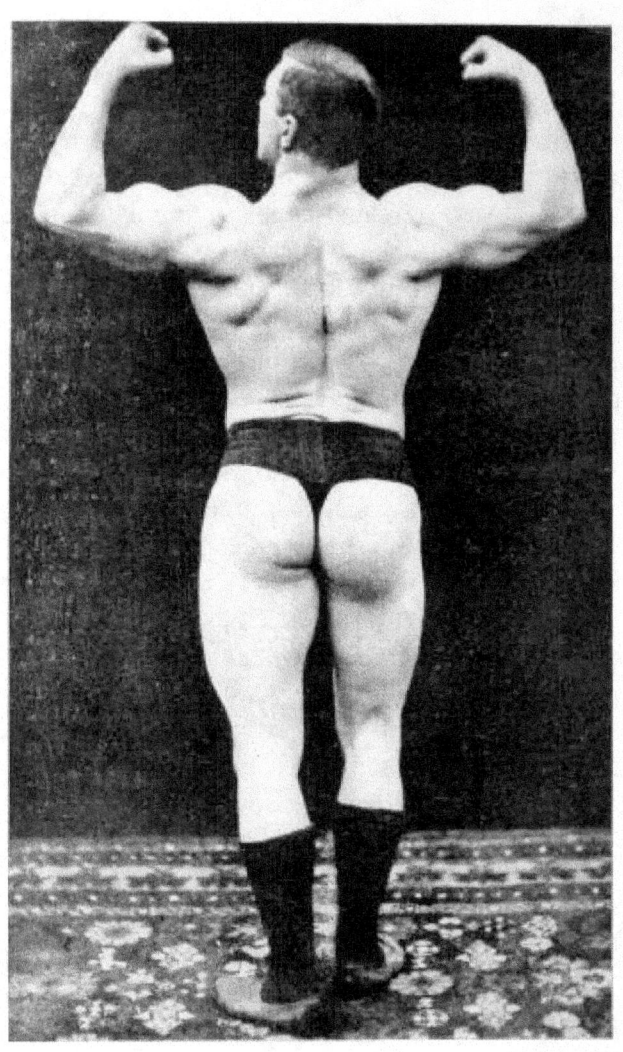

GEORGE HACKENSCHMIDT

His enormous muscles can be likened to a well forged chain—not a single weak spot in his make-up.

If you will observe people's necks, you will see hundreds of different sizes and shapes before you have looked very far. Some are so fleshy in the back that a great many wrinkles can be seen. Others are exceedingly fleshy in front, causing one or two extra chins. Necks that are stringy and appear to have two ugly cords running towards the top of the head in the back are not uncommon. Prominent "Adam's apples" and scrawny, cordy appearances are often seen in the front of the neck.

I have always contended that there is absolutely no excuse for anyone to have a scrawny or ungainly-looking neck, when a few minutes devoted every day to the care and welfare of this part of the body would not only make the pupil feel better, but would change his appearance completely. Double chins can easily be removed with properly applied exercise.

It is not necessary for anyone to develop his neck to the huge proportions of a wrestler's, unless he so desires, but if properly applied exercises are devoted especially to the trapezius muscle in the back and also to the sterno-cleido-mastoid at the sides of the neck, symmetrical lines will make their appearance in a very short space of time.

When exercising the neck, care should be taken not to apply the resistance too vigorously, for sometimes the muscles are over-strained and a kink in the neck is a very unpleasant feeling and lasts for several days. Begin all neck movements slowly.

Neck Movements Should Be Done Slowly in Order to See the Greatest Possible Benefit

Do not perform any of them in a jerky manner, and be careful to avoid strain. The resistance applied behind the head for development of the head in the back should be done in an even, steady manner. The first movement should be much lighter than the second, and the second movement lighter than the third, until about the fifteenth or twentieth count, when the strongest pressure should be applied. By devoting special attention to the back of the neck, you will straighten the appearance of your spine and eliminate the hollows between the occipital bone in the back of the head

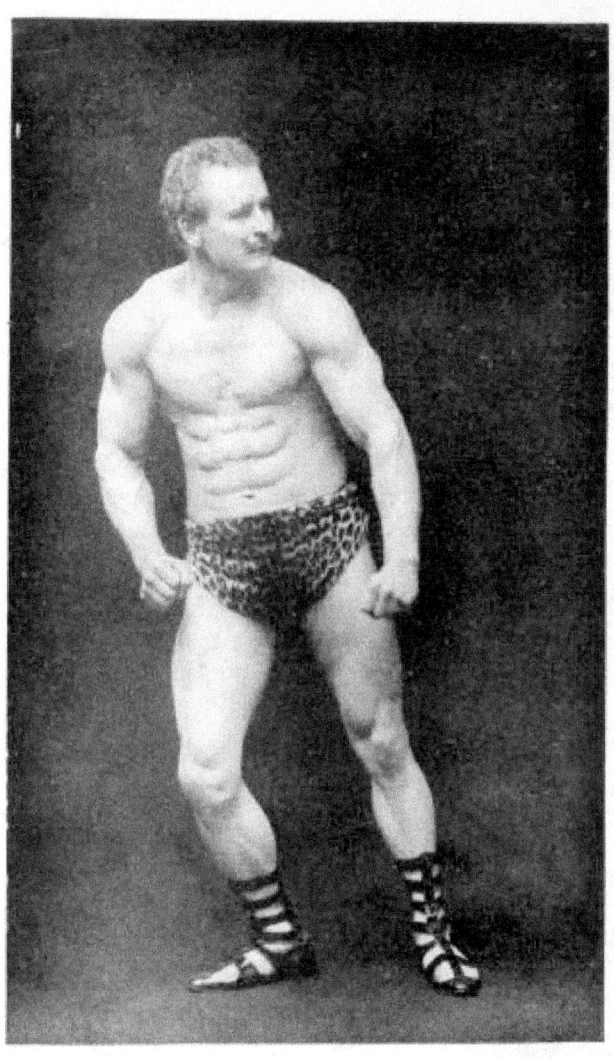

EUGEN SANDOW

An interesting study of the perfect male figure. No matter how he stood or what pose he assumed, Sandow displayed curves from every angle.

and the upper dorsal vertebrae, which gives the appearance of round shoulders. By having the neck developed straight in the back, the appearance of the student will be greatly improved, owing to his erect, military posture. By paying attention also to the sterno-cleido-mastoid muscles, at the sides of the neck, it will help square out the neck and give the straight, athletic lines so commonly noticed in anyone who does a great amount of athletic work.

Modern fashions in collars tend to hide the defects in people's necks. Therefore, the time to look at a neck critically is when people are in bathing suits. Then the real truth comes out. For instance, a neck may look fairly pleasing to the eye with a high collar on, but when the high collar comes off, the neck will be found very defective in the lower part, owing to the poor development of the trapezius muscle. Head-circling, turning and twisting, and bending from side to side are common movements for the neck, and this light work will help greatly, when combined with scientifically applied neck movements, towards a symmetrical development. Performing the wrestler's bridge is also excellent for strength purposes, and will help greatly towards further development.

The Size of the Head Is an Important Factor

The size and shape of the head is an important factor in neck development, as I have said before. A person with a narrow face and a long, narrow head cannot and must not expect to obtain the same size neck as a person whose features are of a bull-dog type; that is, square or round. However, such people need not be discouraged, for their necks can be developed to from 15½ to 16½ inches, depending, of course, upon the height of the individual. A person who has a large head and large features naturally requires a much larger neck to harmonize with the rest of his body than his narrow-type friend. Such individuals can easily acquire necks from 16½ to 18 inches, depending again upon the height of the individual.

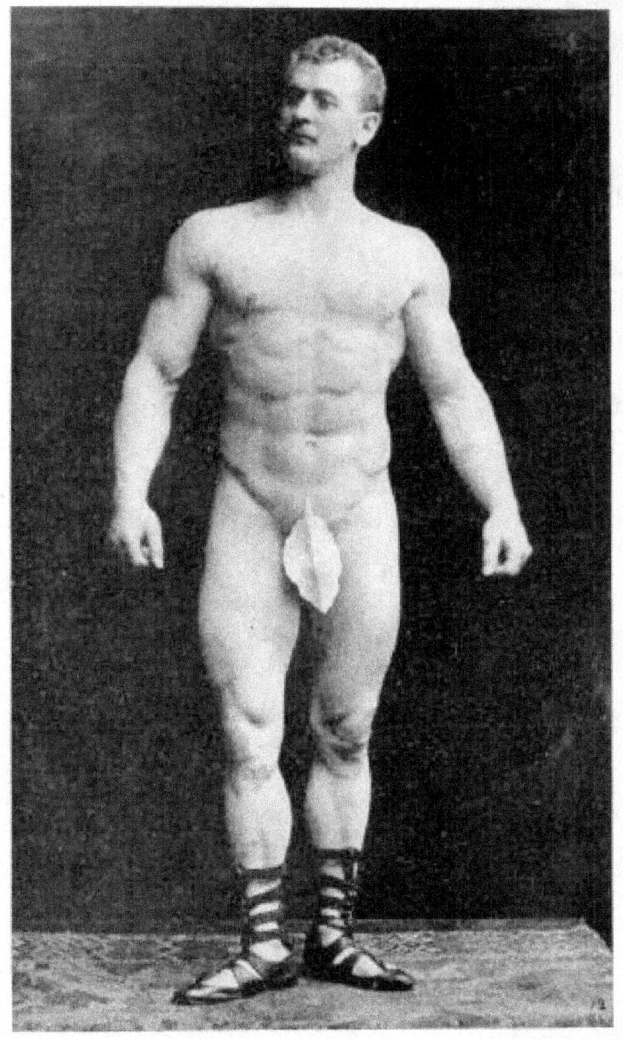

EUGEN SANDOW

Showing how properly developed muscles look in a relaxed state. The reader's attention is called to Sandow's remarkable abdominal development, which even though relaxed, shows prominently in the above photograph.

I have always been thankful that I have developed a strong, muscular neck, for I remember once while bathing in a swimming pool at Long Beach, California, I took a high dive, without any thought as to the depth of the water, and hit the bottom with such force that my arm was thrown against my shoulder and my head hit the bottom so hard and at such an angle, that not only did I have a lump on top of my head the size of a small apple, but my neck and shoulder pained me for many days thereafter. I am positive that if my neck had been weak at this time, it would have snapped. In fact, as every reader of these pages knows, it is not at all uncommon to hear of divers breaking their necks when hitting bottom.

Don't Stock Up Too Heavily on Collars and Shirts

To a person who is desirous of increasing the size of the neck, I suggest that he do not stock up too freely with shirts and collars, for you will find that every week or two you will have to get larger sizes. However, there is no need to fear developing the neck to enormous or ungainly proportions. For when your neck is large enough to suit yourself, all you have to do is to stop development work, and just do light work, such as twisting or turning the neck. This will keep the neck in shape and it will not get any larger.

One of the first places which will tell the condition of an athlete is the back of his neck. When an athlete starts slipping backwards it is usually accompanied by the thinning out of the posterior part of the neck.

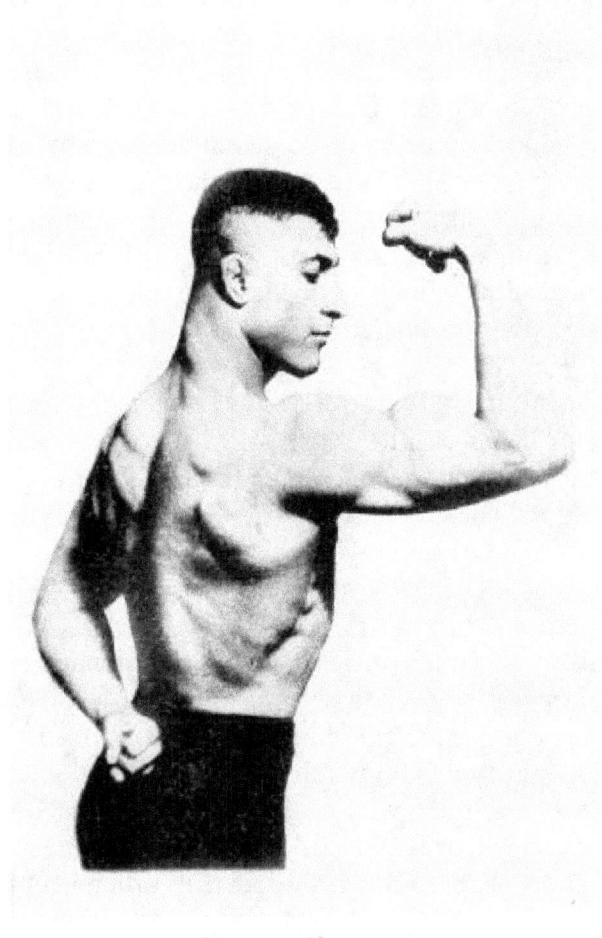

YOUSEFF HOUSANE
Besides having an exceptional muscular development, this 200-pound
wrestler has one of the largest biceps ever seen. It can be likened to a
large baseball.

One of the largest necks I have ever seen on any well-trained athlete was that of George Hackenschmidt, the former world's champion wrestler. Hackenschmidt weighed about 215 pounds, stripped, at the time, with an exceptionally large frame and head. His neck measured 22½ inches. Stanislaus Zbyszko, the noted wrestler, also has a neck that measures well over 20 inches.

However, one of the most remarkable tests of strength I have ever seen put to the neck was when Joseph Vitole, a small, 150-pound athlete, lifted from the floor 550 pounds with his teeth alone. Think of the remarkable bull-dog grip this miniature Hercules possessed at the time of this lift. I particularly noticed the great strain and the manner in which the muscles of the neck bulged outward at the time I saw him make this world's record- breaking lift. Vitole has a neck measuring about 17 inches, but the muscles are of exceptionally fine quality.

Don't Let Your Hair Grow Too Far Down on Your Neck

Now, here's a little secret. If you want to add to the appearance of your neck, do not permit the hair to grow too far down the back, but always keep the hair neatly trimmed. This will not only give you a cleaner appearance from the rear, but it will enable your neck muscles to present their best appearance.

I also want to tell you that by properly applied exercises to the front of the neck, a prominent "Adam's apple" can be made to appear smaller, and all excess flesh under the chin can be eliminated. To my mind nothing is more pleasing to the eye than to see a well-set jaw and chin, backed up by a well-developed neck. You surely know that the way you carry your head makes a wonderful difference in your posture and in your personality. So do not allow your head to drop forward, but endeavor to keep it erect at all times. Remember, that constantly forcing the chin downward will cause wrinkles in the front of the neck, whereas, on the contrary, by constantly holding the chin high in the air, you will have a tendency to cause wrinkles in the back of the neck. My best advice is to study yourself in the mirror, not for the sake of vanity, but for the purpose of looking for improvement and benefiting your appearance.

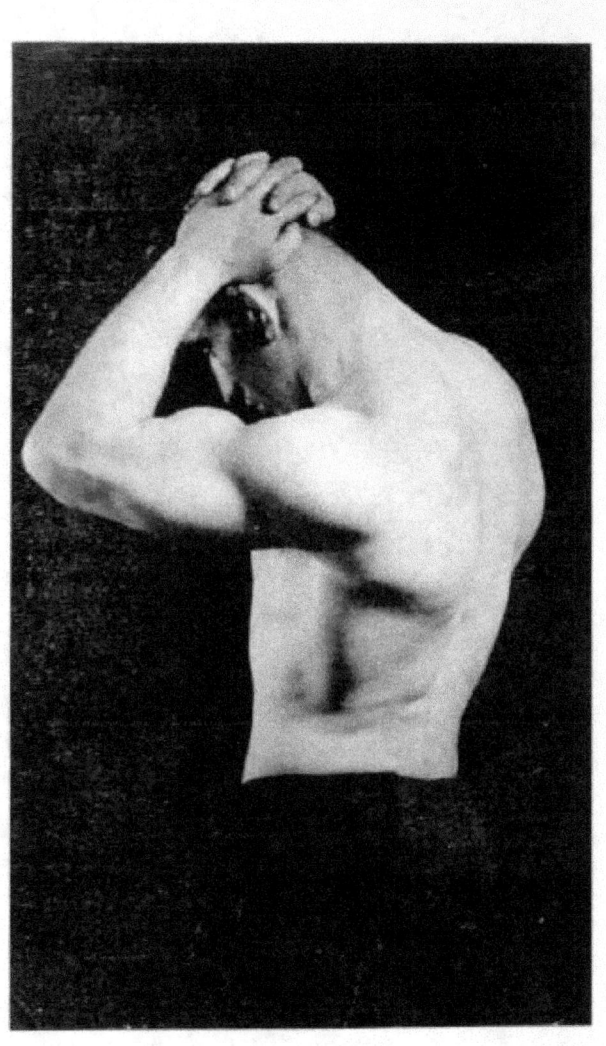

EXERCISE FOR THE NECK

Clasp hands behind head and pull head forward, strongly resisting at the same time with the muscles of the neck. Pull head forward as far as it will go. (See chapter on the neck.)

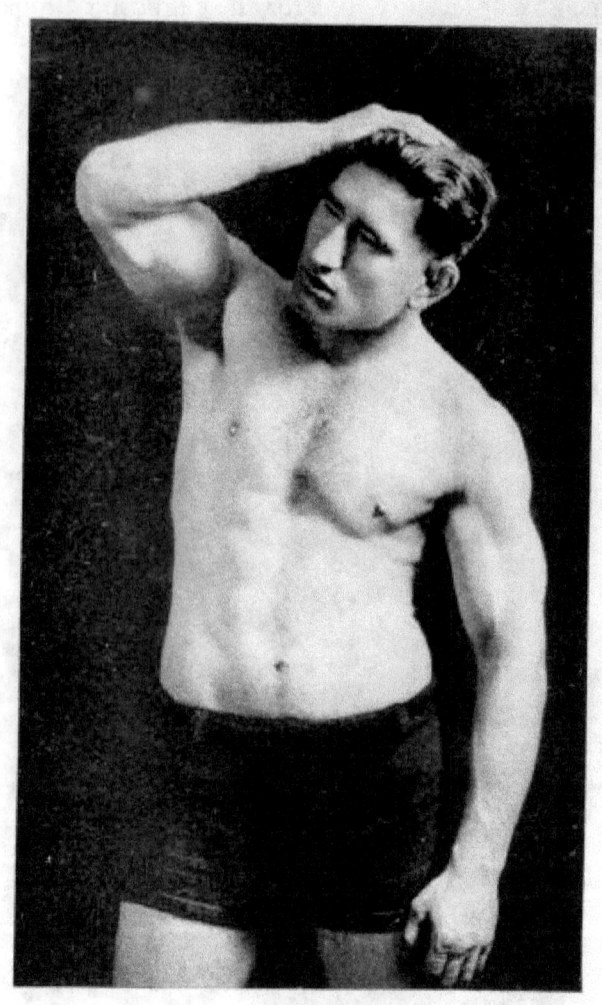

EXERCISE FOR THE NECK

Place hand on side of head and push head to one side, resisting meanwhile with the neck muscles. (See chapter on the neck.)

I may say right here that one reason most singers develop two or more chins is that they are constantly exercising the neck muscles with the lower jaw abnormally
relaxed. It's difficult for them to avoid this, for they really
have to relax these jaw muscles, while at the same time

they are putting a certain amount of tension on the neck muscles.

However, you or any other athlete can avoid this, if you will only bear the following instructions in mind.

Exercises for the Neck

1. Clasp your hands behind the head while sitting or standing erect. Now pull the head forward, strongly resisting at the same time with the muscles of the neck. Make as complete a movement as possible, beginning from an erect posture, and pull the head forward as far as the muscles will allow it to go. This will strengthen and develop the trapezius muscle and give straightness to the back of the neck. Variations to this exercise can be made by first holding the chin in, and again sticking the chin out while performing the movement. (See photograph on page 55.)

2. Place your right hand on the right side of head, and push the head as far as you can to the left, resisting meanwhile with the muscles of the neck. This exercise will develop the sterno-cleido-mastoid muscle and give the neck a square appearance when viewed from the front. Do the same with left hand and push the head to the right. (See photograph on page 56.)

Neither of the two above exercises should be performed less than fifteen counts nor more than twenty-five counts. If the pressure is applied too vigorously, and the muscles become tired in less than fifteen repetitions, there may be a tendency to strain some part of the muscle and cause a very unpleasant kink in the neck. If such a kink is ever experienced, massage the part thoroughly and give the muscle a rest for a few days.

Twisting the head from side to side, bending it forward and backward, bending it from right to left, are excellent movements for limbering up the muscles of the neck, before applying the resistance work mentioned. The neck is one part of the body that is very susceptible to exercise, and if the student is desirous of enlarging this part of the body, with the proper application of resistance, there is no reason why he should not be able to gain an inch or more around the neck in thirty days.

The wrestler's bridge, as I said before, is also of great benefit for strengthening the neck in general. This exercise consists of resting your entire weight on the head and feet alone while the back makes an arch. By raising and lowering the hips while in this position, and by walking a few inches towards the head and back again, the neck will experience quite a variation of movements. A few minutes' daily work in this bridging will greatly help the further progress of neck development. (See photograph opposite.)

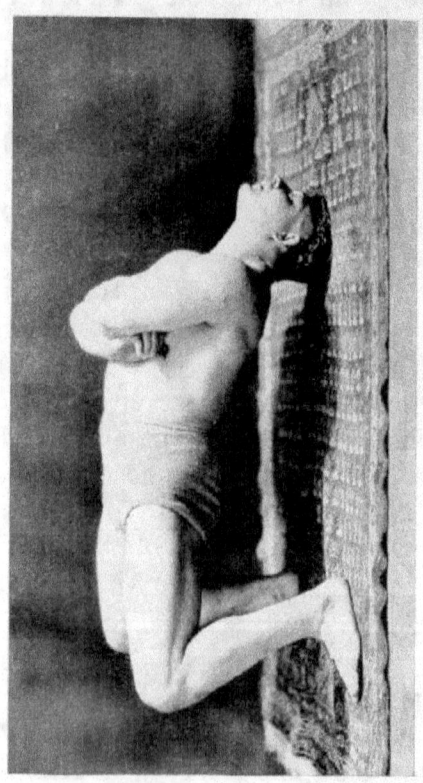

THE WRESTLER'S BRIDGE
A splendid neck exercise practiced by most wrestlers for strengthening the neck muscles. (See chapter on the neck.)

I want to emphasize again that the neck presents a very interesting subject to the student of anatomy. The most ungainly-looking necks are those lacking in development of the trapezius muscle in the back, causing two hideous cords to run upwards into the hair. This is more prominent in thin people when they bend the heads slightly forward. Such cords can be entirely eliminated with proper application of exercises to the back of the neck.

You will frequently find individuals with two or three chins, which can easily be removed by proper application of exercise to the front part of the neck. You will also find prominent "Adam's apples," which can be reduced considerably by developing the muscles of the neck. The person who has never exercised the neck does not have a pleasing contour, especially when without a collar, or when in a bathing or gymnasium costume. Instead of having well-formed, straight, pleasing contour to the muscles, the sterno-cleido-mastoid, and the trapezius seem to grow inward at the bottom of the neck, causing the neck to have a smaller appearance at the bottom than at the top, when on the contrary the neck should be larger at the bottom than at the top.

Professional wrestlers' necks, although oftentimes over-developed, have excellent contour, and no matter which way their heads are turned, or carried, they present a pleasing appearance. Yet anyone can obtain the same contour in the neck which professional wrestlers have, without the over-development which gives the bulllike appearance. A well-developed neck means an increased blood supply to the brain.

This gives the owner a clearer thinking capacity, owing to the enlargement of the veins and arteries inside of the neck.

All neck exercises, as I said before, should be per-formed from fifteen to twenty-five counts. Any work that is more vigorous and tires the muscles with a less number of repetitions than this, will be apt to strain the ligaments and muscles, so that painful results might follow. You must not force the development of the neck as vigorously as you would the arms. Such strenuous measures, however, are unnecessary; for, as I have previously stated, the neck responds rapidly to properly applied activity. At about the twentieth count, the amount of resistance applied to the neck should cause the muscles to begin to ache, so that by the twenty-fifth repetition, the aching point should cause a student to naturally discontinue.

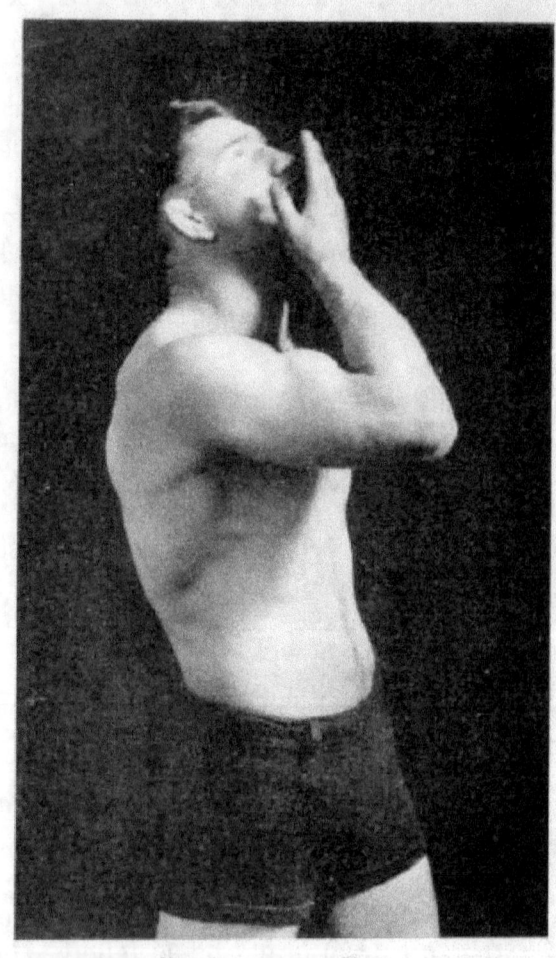

EXERCISE FOR THE NECK

Place hand on chin and push head backwards, resisting strongly with the neck muscles. (See chapter on the neck.)

I wish to make it very clear that I consider the development of the neck of very great importance. So do not get the idea into your head that you should favor or specialize in the development of your arms, shoulders and chest. In all my work I aim at a perfect, symmetrical development, and, in my opinion, there is nothing of greater importance in physical development than the development of the muscles of your neck.

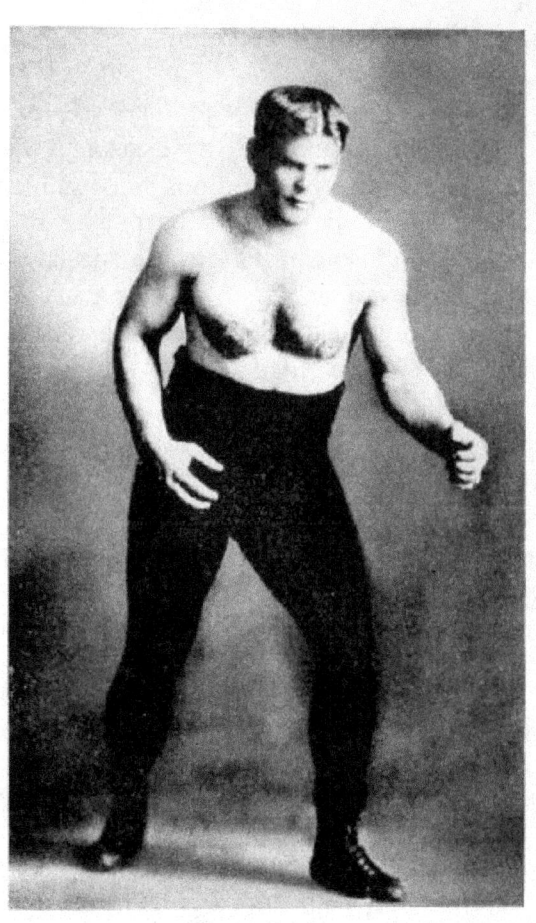

FRANK GOTCH

The late world's champion wrestler. A naturally strong, stocky man whose muscles acted in perfect co-ordination. His strength was likened to a grizzly's.

Chapter IV
The Shoulders and Their Development

SOME time ago a husky-looking chap came to me for physical examination and advice. I had the young fellow strip and put him through a few moderately severe exercises, to determine what condition he was in.

I found he was very well qualified in most of the strength tests, with the exception of the "push up" and certain other exercises that required superior development of the deltoids.

His arms, chest and legs were very well developed, but it was evident to myself and my assistants that this man hadn't done any really conscientious work on his shoulders.

I pointed out his defect, and he put himself under my care, with the purpose of taking some special exercises for the muscles that were lacking in development. I took careful measurements, and also several photographs- front, back and side views—and filed them away for subsequent comparison.

The young fellow worked faithfully under my direction for several months. At the expiration of that time, he came back to see me and report progress. You wouldn't believe that such a change could be wrought in a chap who was originally a pretty husky, presentable looking individual. For the improvement was simply wonderful. He had muscles that weren't apparent at all when I first examined him. His tests showed about 58 per cent, increase in deltoid strength and endurance, and he was a perfect picture of manhood.

So, I say that the neglect of this one muscle often shows a lack of condition in an athlete, and this one muscle is the deltoid or shoulder muscle. When the deltoids are full, round, thick and bulging, it signifies the athlete is in splendid shape. But when they become flat and flabby, and the back becomes the broadest part of the body, then it is significant that the athlete is far from being in good condition.

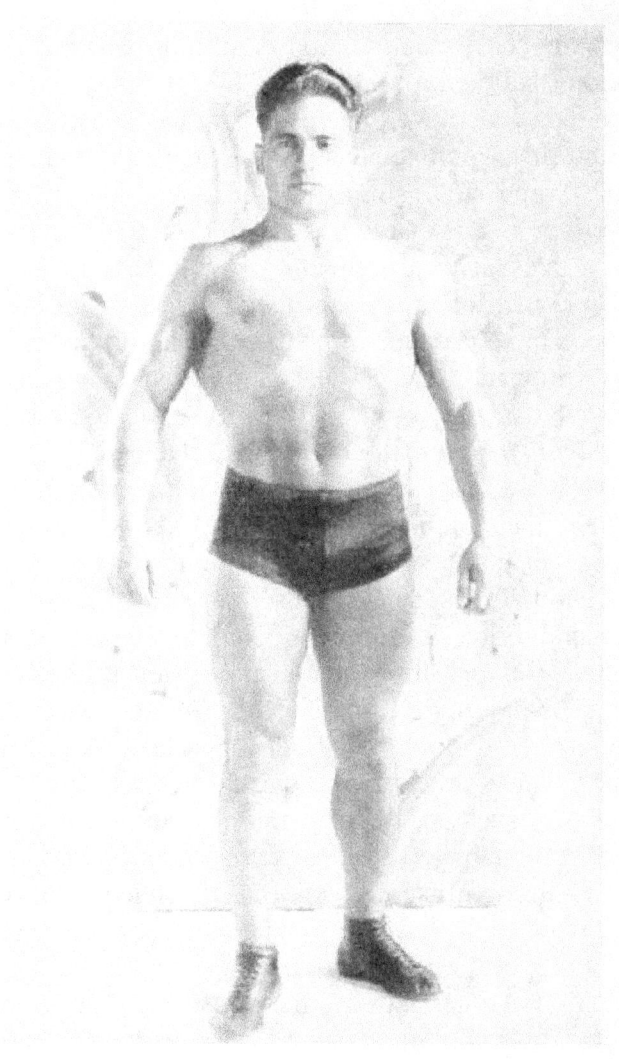

JIM LONDOS

A stocky strong man whose muscles are smooth yet possess bulk. His very pose suggests vitality.

The Deltoid Prime of Life

The deltoid or shoulder muscles are most prominent between the ages of twenty and thirty. It is then that the cords and inner fibers show themselves to best advantage. But as a rule, after thirty years of age, a man's shoulders, providing he keeps in good condition, become somewhat thicker and less prominent. After the age of forty, the shoulders can never again regain the same contour. Of course, if an individual has done but little training he can make wonderful gains after the age of forty, but I am referring in this paragraph to the already trained athlete who values his measurements and muscle contour.

One inch of muscle on the shoulder makes a vast difference in appearance in breadth. I want to make this point very emphatic, as I wish to impress upon young men, particularly, the dangers of delay and procrastination, if they ever want to really build themselves up.

Now, in order to develop the shoulders to a maximum degree, the anterior and posterior deltoids must be exercised in co-operation with the external or side portion. The action of the deltoid muscle is to lift the arm from the side and bring it upwards until it "is parallel with the ground. Beyond this point further action is assisted by the trapezius muscle. It is practically impossible for anyone to exercise the deltoid or shoulder muscle without getting the trapezius, back and arm muscles to work as well.

Well-developed deltoids are very pleasing to look at and set the athlete off considerably. Boxing, bag-punching or any form of exercise that has a tendency to swing the shoulders, will develop the deltoid muscles. However, direct application can be had by systematic exercising, including the raising of the arms forward, sideways or backwards with a resistance to work against. In this manner much heavier shoulder muscles can be developed than in the mere swinging of the arms, as in boxing or bag-punching, and this was exactly what I developed in the young man of whom I spoke earlier in this chapter.

When the Tailor Made the Man

Years ago when men's styles featured broad shoulders, the weak individual depended entirely upon the tailor to make him broader. However, the present-day styles do not contemplate padding in the shoulders. Therefore to possess an athletic appearance, everyone must devote special training to the deltoid muscles, in order to broaden the shoulders and add to his general appearance.

The size of the bones again plays an important part in the general width of anyone's shoulders. The small-framed individual cannot expect to become as broad-shouldered as one who possesses a large framework, but, nevertheless, the small-boned man can broaden his shoulders a few inches by devoting attention to the deltoid muscle.

As a rule, horizontal bar and ring performers have exceptionally developed shoulder muscles. The same can be found in weight lifters. However, anyone can strengthen and develop the deltoid muscle to the maximum by scientifically and systematically applied exercise.

The shoulder muscles, as a rule, become tired quicker than any other part of your body when doing competitive work. This can be clearly illustrated when swimming. If your wind is in excellent condition, you will find the shoulders will usually be first affected by the continual efforts.

There is one other matter of which I wish to speak, and which I consider most important, especially to those who wish to possess a really symmetrical development. I urgently recommend a great deal of attention to the posterior deltoid, as well as the external fibers. If too much effort is given to the anterior deltoid, it will have a tendency to make one appear somewhat round-shouldered.

I have seen many an otherwise splendid physique marred by the failure to observe this little point.

How to Overcome Round Shoulders

Round shoulders may rightly be considered one of the worst handicaps to anyone who aspires to physical perfection. And they are quite inexcusable. Such a man is downright lazy or indifferent about his appearance.

One of the finest exercises for overcoming round shoulders is to bring the arms from a front position parallel with the floor to a position as far back as they are capable of going; keeping them parallel at all times, and working against a powerful resistance. Then, again, the shoulders should be brought back as far as possible after the completion of each exercise period, in order to shorten the muscles of the back. This will offset the tendency of the shoulders to drop forward after you have given them vigorous exercise.

Measuring the Shoulders

A person whose shoulders measure more than 18 inches can be considered quite broad. I have known in some cases, however, of remarkably developed athletes, where the shoulders measured more than 24 inches across. Perhaps you may not know the proper way of measuring the shoulders. I have yet to find many who do.

The simple method of measuring the shoulders is by having someone place two sticks, rods or rulers at the end of each shoulder, parallel with each other. Then the measurement should be taken in between these sticks. If you attempt to measure your shoulders by placing the tape across the front or behind the back, you will not get an accurate measurement. Instead, you may find yourself one or two inches broader than you really are.

How to Obtain Quickest Results

The larger the deltoids become the better they set off the arms. The best way to develop these muscles is to raise the arms forward, sideways, and backwards, to the height of the shoulder, all the while working against a resistance. Whether this resistance be in the form of an adjustable dumb-bell, elastic exerciser or other apparatus, the resistance should be progressive, and increased each week as the shoulders become stronger.

In order to obtain the quickest results, the repetitions should not exceed from ten to fifteen counts. If the student exercises so vigorously as to make it impossible for him to do more than five or six repetitions, he is using up his strength too rapidly and retards his development.

I have found from experience that the best results can be obtained for the shoulders by carrying the repetitions to over ten and less than fifteen counts. However, if the muscles do not begin to ache a little at the fifteenth repetition, the pupil should work against a stronger resistance. If you perform light work, and it takes, for example, thirty-five to fifty repetitions before the deltoids reach their aching point, you can tell the work is too light for you. Of course, some progress can be made, so far as endurance and development is concerned, by performing these lighter movements. But no great degree of deltoid development can be reached unless you work against resistance strong enough to tire the muscles within fifteen repetitions. You must progress each week by adding more resistance to the work, providing, of course, it becomes easier to do fifteen counts in the exercise than it did the previous week.

I am not an advocate of resistance movements, neither am I against them. Resistance movements are all right for bringing the muscles out for posing or photographic purposes, but they are inferior to movements where artificial resistance is used, because of the fact that while performing resistance work, the pupil is apt to resume the resistance with the mind wandering, and also by giving too much attention to his feelings. There is also a tendency to discover easier methods of performing the exercises, and such discoveries are fatal to physical progress.

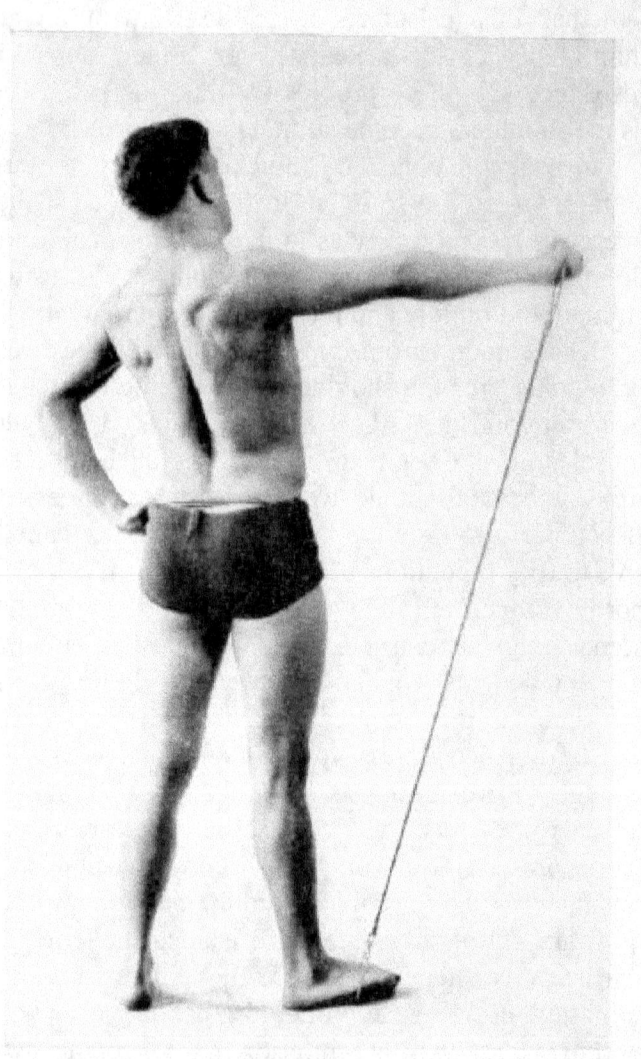

EXERCISE FOR THE SHOULDERS

Raise arm sideways to height of shoulder, working against a resistance. This movement will broaden the shoulders. (See chapter on the shoulders.)

Some Exercises for Your Shoulders

1. Stand erect; raise the arms with a weight or exerciser forward until they are parallel with the floor and at the height of the shoulder. Now lower and repeat. This will develop the anterior deltoid. If the palm of hand is kept facing downward, the supinator muscles of the forearm are also benefited considerably.

2. Raise the arm sideways, until the arm is parallel with the floor, and at the height of the shoulders; keep palm down. This movement will develop the external head of the deltoid and broaden the shoulders, at the same time benefiting the external head of the triceps.

3. Raise arm backwards as far as possible. This movement is for the posterior deltoid and the upper back muscles as well. If the arm is kept rigid while performing this movement, the internal head of the triceps receives considerable work. By paying attention to the anterior and the posterior parts of the deltoid muscle, the shoulder will become thicker and will have more depth.

It is not uncommon to see individuals with wide shoulders whose external deltoids are remarkably developed, but who are sadly lacking in the anterior and posterior sections of this muscle, thus giving them a thin appearance.

When the deltoid is properly developed, there are a series of fibers or digitations faintly showing at the external portion. These fibers give an excellent appearance to the deltoids under proper lighting. With the posterior deltoid properly developed, the fleshy lumps will help greatly to make the back straight and set off the roundness of the back.

If you are really interested in bringing out all the fine points in your physique I strongly urge you to pay a great deal of attention to the development of your deltoids, for they certainly contribute in a great way toward making up the ideal figure of a man. And this is what we all want to do.

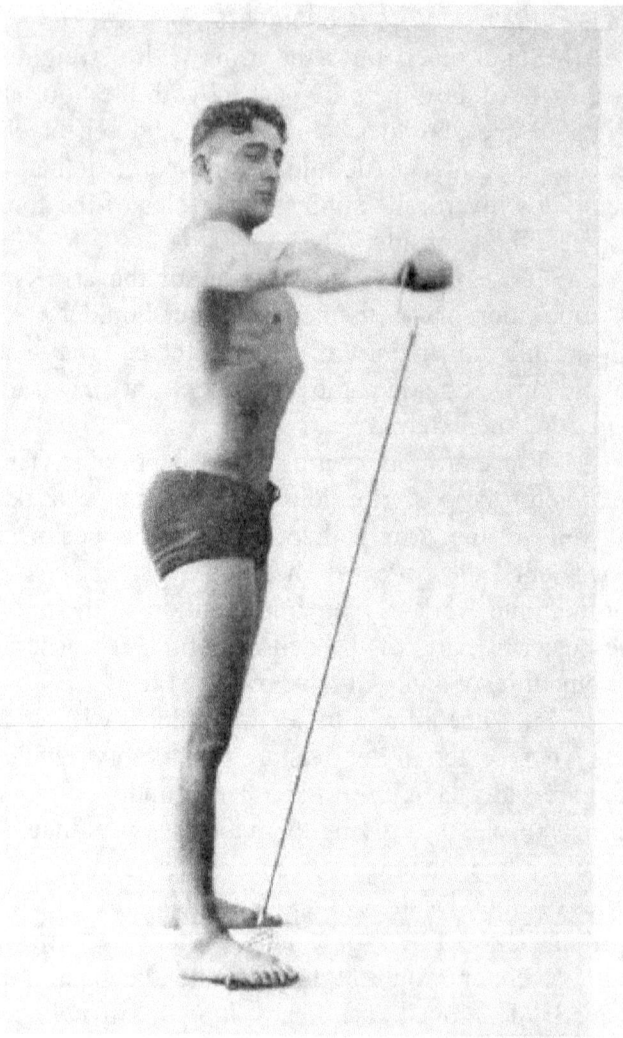

EXERCISE FOR THE SHOULDERS

Raise arm forward to the height of shoulder, working against a resistance. This exercise will develop the front part of deltoid muscle. (See chapter on the shoulders.)

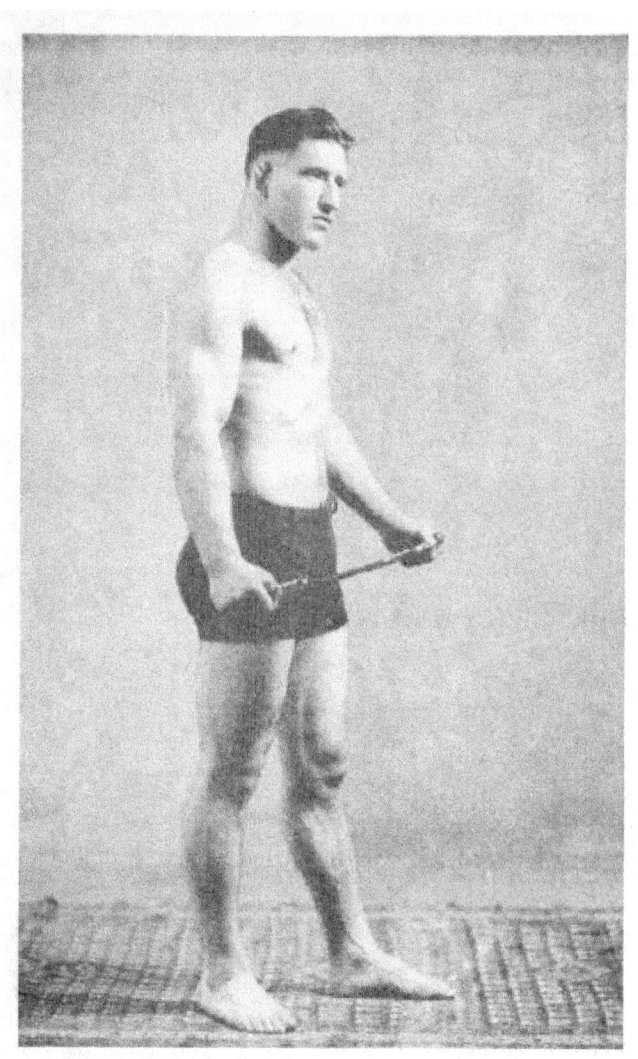

EXERCISE FOR THE SHOULDERS
Hold the exercises with arms straight as shown above.

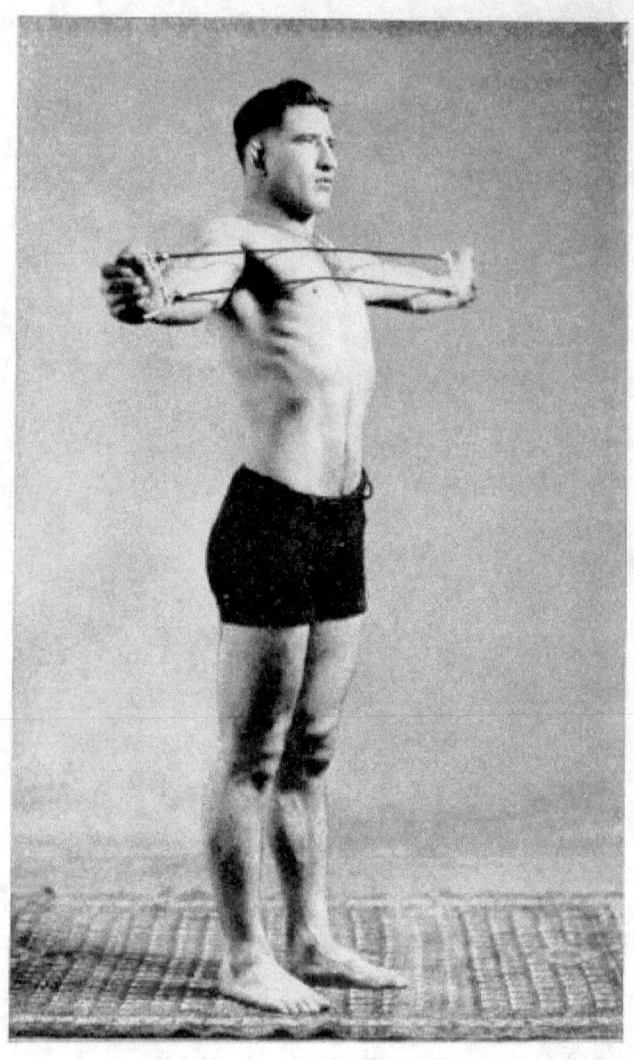

EXERCISE FOR THE SHOULDERS

*Then raise both arms sideways to height of shoulders while stretch-
ing the exerciser apart. (See chapter on the shoulders.)*

Chapter V
The Perfect Back and How to Develop It

THE muscles of the back are undoubtedly the most interesting sets of muscles in the body, owing both to their remarkable formation and to their great number. Even though everyone's muscles have the same origin and insertion, still the formation of back developments differ greatly. The majority of backs not only have a stoop-shouldered effect, but they are practically flat in appearance, owing to the lack of proper muscular development. A well-muscled back should have quite a cavity running from the base of the neck downward towards the hips, and this cavity is harmoniously situated between well-rounded muscles.

It is almost impossible to neglect the shoulders and back if you perform arm work, and if the proper exercises are indulged in, the back and shoulders are worked in co-ordination with the arms. This is the way a person should exercise the muscles—in groups. With proper attention paid to the back muscles, the student need have little fear of ever becoming stoop-shouldered, although if the back is over-developed, there will be a tendency to round shoulders.

This can be eliminated by devoting a little time after each drill to straightening up exercises, such as clasping the hands behind the hips with arms stiff, and forcing the shoulders back as far as possible, until the shoulder blades touch. This should be performed after each drill, and repeated quite a number of times, as it will shorten the back muscles and lengthen the pectorals of the chest, which draw the shoulders forward.

The most prominent muscle of the back is the latissimus dorsi. This muscle covers almost the entire sides and the back, from the waist to the armpits, and inserts itself along the spinous processes of the fifth and sixth thoracic and the lumbar vertebrae. This muscle can be developed to enormous proportions. The greater it is developed the more slant the individual possesses from the arm pits to the waist, and the broader his back becomes, not to speak of the pleasing appearance it presents in the form of beautiful, rolling muscles.

How the Back Muscles Are Developed

The latissimus dorsi muscle is developed by the constant pulling of the arms from an overhead position downward, whether this is accomplished in a forward movement or a side movement. Chinning the bar is another great exercise for this muscle. Any movement is helpful that tends to bring the arms downward, whether lifting a heavy weight from the floor while stooping forward and coming to an erect position, or whether the arms are worked against a strong resistance from an overhead start. The action is practically the same in either case.

The latissimus dorsi muscle is usually of great prominence in professional athletes, for no one is satisfied with his appearance until he has attained somewhere near the maximum proportions in this muscle. Until this muscle has been highly developed, the pupil must not expect to be as powerful or as symmetrically developed as he will become after devoting consistent attention to his back. I have seen almost unbelievable proportions in this muscle on some prominent strong men. When the muscle has been developed to its maximum equally on each side, it can be tensed so as to make the back broader in appearance than the entire width of the shoulders.

The trapezius muscle, covering the upper back on each side of the neck and giving the slant from the neck to the shoulders, is another important muscle that requires considerable attention. When highly developed it greatly improves the athlete's appearance. This muscle is used in shrugging the shoulders. It also assists in raising the shoulders and arms upward, after they pass a horizontal position.

It is one of the first muscles of a weak individual which tires as a result of carrying a heavy suit case. The constant lifting of heavy objects from the floor in standing erect with the arms at the sides will develop this muscle. When properly developed and when the muscles of the back are tensed for display, these muscles have the appearance of a W in the center of the back. These muscles are also developed by the constant contraction of the shoulders when the pupil endeavors to swing the arms backwards, working against a resistance, such as a heavy tensioned chest expander. If these two major muscles of the back work in co-ordination, not only an interesting muscular display can be accomplished, but the owner will be able to perform feats of strength that will be impossible for the average properly trained athlete.

The Center of Your Nervous Energy

The center of the nervous system which contains most of your energy, lies in the small of the back. Therefore, if you are constantly bending and stooping forward, backward and sideways, preferably against a strong resistance of some kind, you will acquire a powerful back that will stimulate the nervous system, as well as eliminate all backaches and tired feelings that usually manifest themselves in this region.

The first signs of weakness and run-down condition usually appear in the small of the back. This causes pain or stiffness in that portion of the body. However, a well-trained athlete need have little fear of these common ailments. For, if the student who is past middle age and is beginning to slip backwards, will devote a little attention to this part of his body, not only will he find his health improving, but also his vitality will be ever on the increase, instead of on the down-hill grade.

How to Get the Best Results with Back Muscle Concentration

Although it is difficult to exercise the arms and shoulders without giving the back plenty of work at the same time, still the exercise that the back receives when the movements are applied directly to the arms or shoulders, does not influence the back muscles as directly as if the pupil concentrated only upon the muscle or groups of muscles he desires to develop. Therefore, in order to produce the best results and the most rapid progress for the muscles of the back, concentration and direct application must be placed on this part.

As the latissimus dorsi is the largest muscle of the back, naturally the student will notice the progress of this muscle sooner than other muscles of the back. Although swimming is about the best exercise calling into play the latissimus dorsi muscle, still the lightness of the movements will not produce as quick results for this muscle as heavier exercise. Chinning the bar is a much heavier exercise for this muscle than is swimming. Consequently the student will progress more rapidly and obtain more of a slant from his armpits to his waist through the practice of chinning than he will from swimming. Rope climbing is of special benefit to this latissimus dorsi muscle, as also is the lifting of a heavy weight from the floor. This latter should be done while stooping forward and keeping the knees stiff, and raising the weight to the height of the waistline and lowering it again.

And, again, the arms may be brought downward and backward from a forward position, or brought downward from a side position, as both movements hit this muscle directly. The greater the resistance in this movement, the quicker the results.

Contracting the Latissimus Dorsi Muscles for Show Purposes

Most athletes are quite conscious of this latissimus dorsi muscle and as a result they usually keep it contracted when they are appearing before the public. Although contraction of this muscle shows its size to advantage, nevertheless, the muscle is more pleasing to the eye when relaxed, for it is in this condition that the harmonious curves express themselves.

I have found from experience and observation that the latissimus dorsi muscle is about the easiest muscle to develop, excepting, perhaps, the neck muscles. Therefore, if the student will devote systematic exercise to the betterment of this splendid muscle of the back, he will very soon appreciate more fully the values of scientifically applied physical culture. With this muscle developed to the maximum degree, the differences in chest measurement from contracted to expanded chest will startle the average person. Although this is not true of lung expansion, nevertheless the contraction of the muscles constitutes a standard in chest expanded measurements.

I have seen professional strong men whose expansion with the aid of the latissimus dorsi muscle and other muscles made a difference of over 20 inches from the contracted chest measurement to the fully expanded measurement. As a matter of curiosity, I measured my own chest, while writing this chapter, and found a difference of 14½ inches from the contracted measurement to the complete inhalation combined with muscular expansion.

Some Exercises for the Latissimus Dorsi

EXERCISE 1. Pick up weight from the floor in front of you by stooping over without bending the knees. Raise the weight to the height of the waistline and lower.

EXERCISE 2. Chin the bar, first with hands close together and later with hands wide apart. Keep palms of hands facing you. Do the same exercise with the palms of the hands turned away from you.

EXERCISE 3. Stand sideways to the wall and hold the exerciser at arm's length. Bring the exerciser downward to the side while keeping arms stiff. Do the same with the other arm.

It is very difficult to find exercises that will tire the latissimus dorsi muscle within ten repetitions, for if the resistance is too strong, there is a tendency for the arms or shoulders to tire first. I have found that the best results are obtained by having sufficient resistance to tire this muscle in about fifteen counts. If you are able to perform more than twenty repetitions in exercising this muscle, the work is too light for you and you must work against a stronger resistance, or use heavier weights, as with the deltoid and other muscles.

The Trapezius Muscle of the Back

If this muscle is over-developed, it will have a tendency to make the individual appear somewhat round- shouldered when viewed from the front or from the side, owing to the huge formation of the upper part, bulging on the upper back between the neck and the shoulders. The student should take great care in practicing straightening-up exercises after each period spent in training this muscle, to shorten it, and get it in the habit of assuming an erect carriage.

I am a great believer in exercising the muscles in groups as much as possible, especially those of the back, for if the pupil endeavors to exercise each muscle individually, he will soon tire from lack of vitality. You have only a certain amount of energy to expend at each drill; therefore, you should exercise systematically, so as to tire as many muscles with each movement as possible, thereby conserving your energy and saving time.

There is hardly any need for the pupil to devote special exercise to the small of the back, providing he performs the exercise of picking up weights from the floor to the height of the waist. This movement gives direct play upon the latissimus dorsi and at the same time hits the muscles of the small of the back directly. Therefore, in this movement, you are tiring both the latissimus dorsi muscles and the various muscles in the lumbar region. You also put great stress upon the trapezius muscle.

A similar example can be illustrated when applying exercise to this trapezius muscle. By moving the arms sideways and upwards, or from forward to backwards while the arms are parallel with the floor, and while working against a heavy resistance, the deltoid and trapezius muscles can be worked in unison, and thereby tired together.

I do not believe in the concentration of your work on individual muscles, unless the student is particularly desirous of developing a certain muscle at the expense of others. If, for example, the student is lacking in latissimus dorsi development and has good trapezius muscles, and good deltoids, then, in that case, it will be advisable for him to exercise the latissimus dorsi muscles individually, until they are developed in proportion with the surrounding muscles.

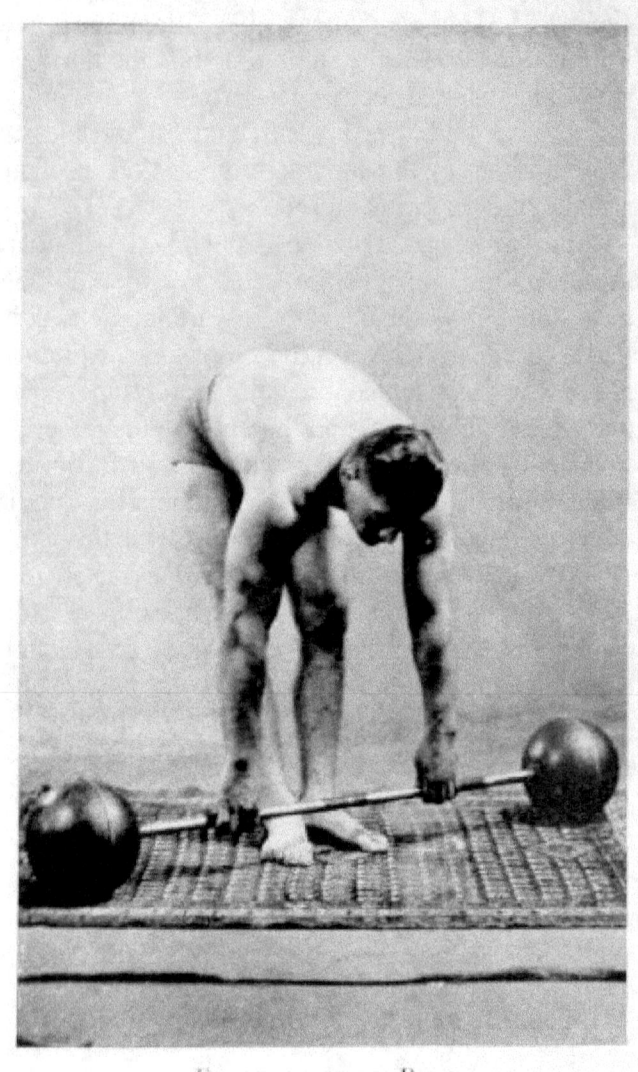

EXERCISE FOR THE BACK

Grasp bar-bell as shown above, while keeping both arms and legs stiff.

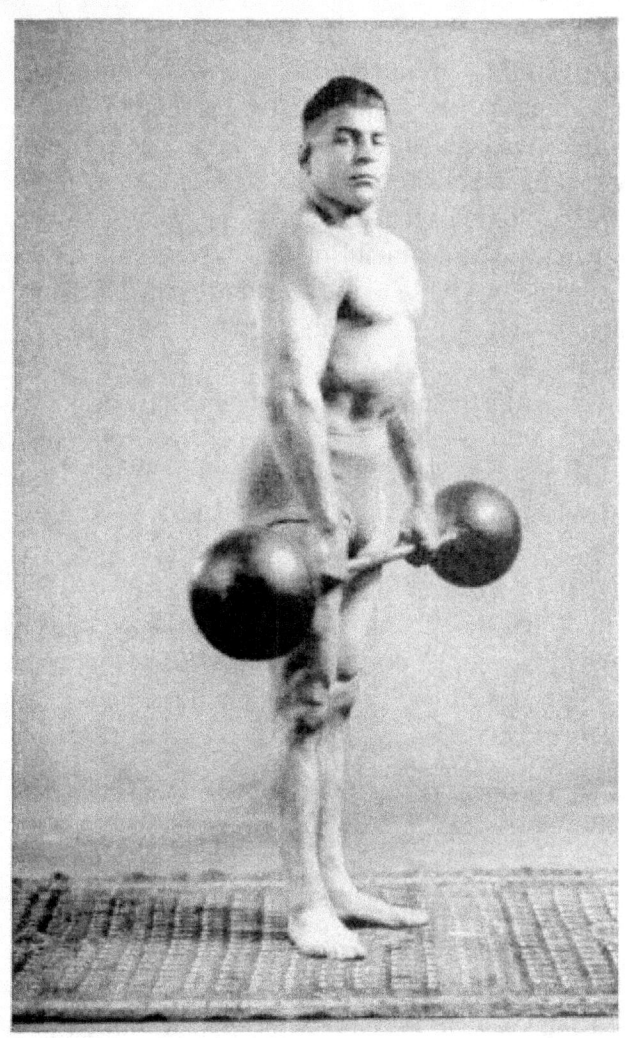

EXERCISE FOR THE BACK
Then come to erect position and repeat. (See chapter on the back.)

Study Others

I have always been an enthusiast in muscular development and symmetrical physiques. Therefore, it may not seem strange if I say that I really believe a highly developed and symmetrically built man is even more pleasing to look at than a beautifully formed woman. The contrast is so great. Even though a beautifully formed woman soothes the eye, nevertheless, I myself would rather study the rippling muscles of a professional athlete than I would the contour of the female form. I have always been this way, and I ascribe this close observation and study of muscular development to the enthusiasm that has stimulated me to make the progress I have in the world of physical culture.

Let your feeling be more than one of admiration when studying the physiques of others. Let it grip your heart and soul and it will eventually change you. Just as a weaker character is influenced by a stronger, so your physical welfare can be influenced by some athlete who is superior to you physically.

The Value of an Ideal

Many years ago I made the acquaintance of one of America's most highly developed athletes, by the name of Adolph Nordquest. I had seen this remarkable man perform on numerous occasions, and had always admired his amazing muscles and remarkable strength. I used to study him for hours, both in admiration and criticism, and I do not think I ever found a flaw in his make-up. I asked him once to tell me what stimulated him to obtain his goal. Did anyone influence him, or what was his ideal in development?

He very quickly told me that Eugen Sandow always was his ideal, and he tried to resemble him in every way possible. He even adopted at one time the professional nom de plume of "Young Sandow," and I must say his physique greatly resembled the original Eugen Sandow's physique.

When in my youth, I, too, had ideals which I followed. Although I did not develop myself along the same lines as these men, nevertheless, I have succeeded far better than might have been expected. So, whether the student adopts an ideal from the person or from the photograph of any certain athlete or strong man, and even though he does not develop himself to this perfection and resemblance, he may obtain strength and muscles that will greatly exceed his expectations.

Observe Your Back Carefully

One of the most common tendencies on the part of the student of physical culture is to devote more attention to the front part of the body than to the back. This is perfectly natural, owing to the fact that a person cannot see his back, but is constantly looking at his front view in the mirror, and sees his defects and improvements in the front only. Systematically applied exercises must be done for the parts hidden from your face as well.

If you turn your back to the mirror and look through a small hand mirror placed in front of you, you will be able to get a better conception of the formation of the back muscles. If you stand under a good light it will enable you to study them better, and also look for defects. You must study your body. I advise daily mirror gazing for this purpose. You need not make this period one of admiration, but simply study the formation and the movements of your muscles, and look wholly for defects—nothing else. Let the admiration come from others.

A Very Important Mirror Tip

While I am on this subject, I might mention that if you desire to see yourself as others see you, and at the same distance as others would be when looking at you, always remember that when you face a full-length mirror, your reflection is twice the distance between you and the mirror. Therefore, you see yourself as others would see you if standing that distance away from you.

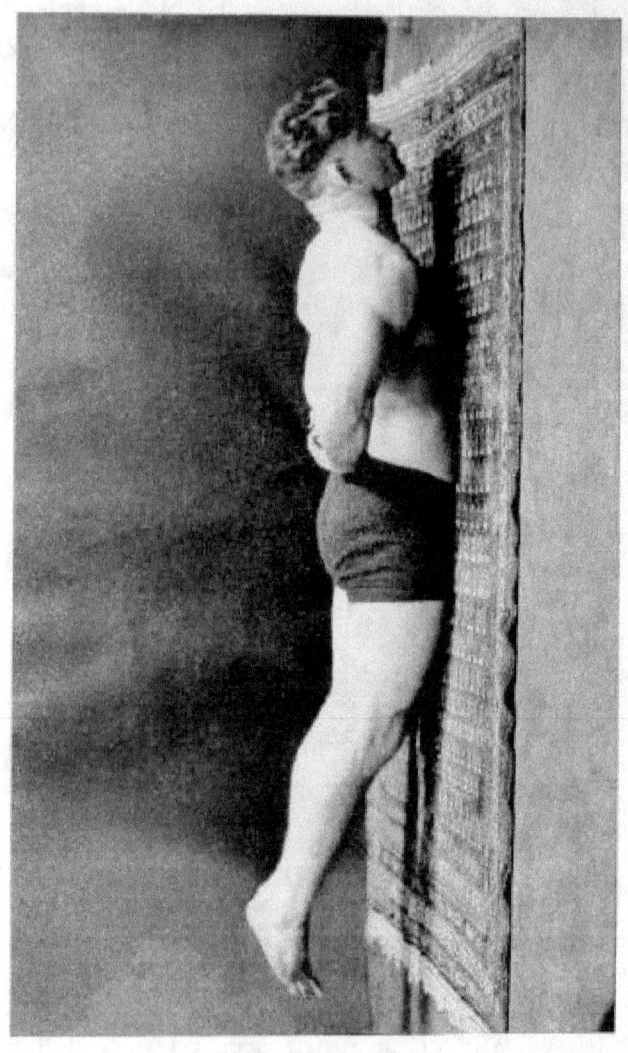

EXERCISE FOR THE BACK

Lie on floor on abdomen and interlace hands behind hips. Then raise legs upwards, keeping knees stiff. To make this exercise harder, raise shoulders and head upwards, while raising legs at same time. (See chapter on the back.)

To make things clearer: if you stand 10 feet away from your mirror, your reflection will be as it actually appears 20 feet away from you. Therefore, you see yourself as someone else would see you—20 feet away. Naturally, in looking at your reflection, you endeavor to look your best. This is human nature. It is like being fitted for a suit of clothes. You have a tendency to stand erect, not mainly to help your tailor, but because you enjoy seeing yourself always at your best. Then when the clothes come from the tailor, they do not always fit you as perfectly as you expect them to, because unless you stand erect and assume your best posture, a few wrinkles in the material will develop.

The same thing applies when studying your body in the mirror. If you always look at yourself at your best, you will have to be continually self-conscious when appearing before others, whether in a gymnasium costume or bathing suit, in order to look the same as you last saw yourself. Therefore, simply stand straight, but relaxed, when studying your body in the mirror, for this is how others will see you. If you are anything but relaxed at all times, not only will you develop considerable self- consciousness, but you will find it a very tedious and tiresome undertaking.

The only thing you should be conscious of at all times is an erect posture. Therefore, if you will constantly assume this posture, so as to avoid a hollow chest and round shoulders, gradually you will form the habit of sitting, standing and walking erect at all times. It will even be difficult for you to assume anything except a proper position.

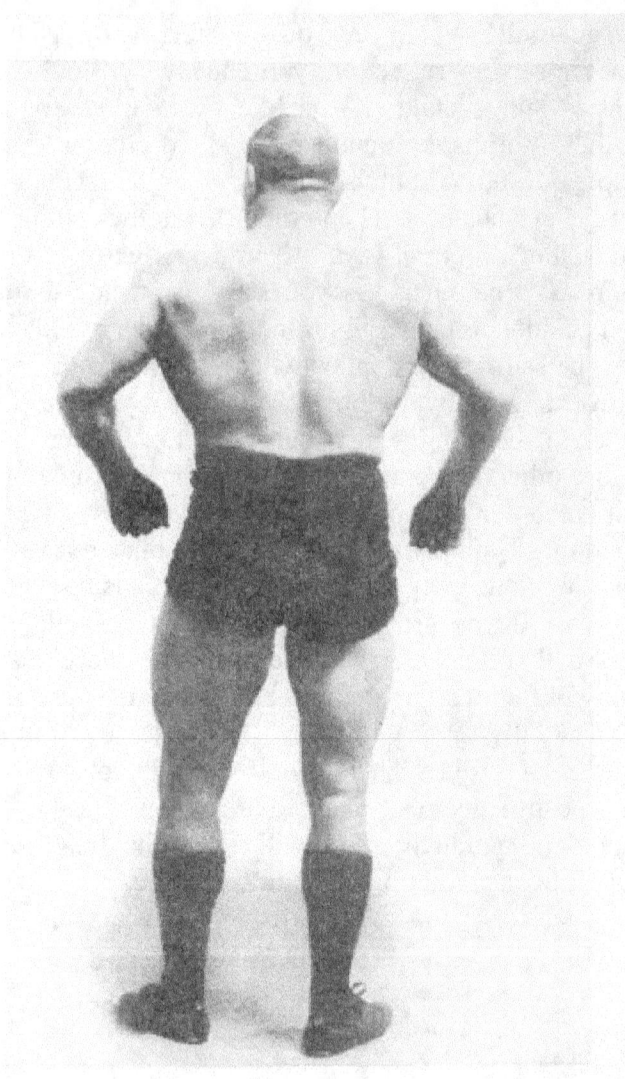

GEORGE HACKENSCHMIDT
Showing the remarkable development of the latissimus dorsi muscle, which when flexed adds considerable breadth to the back.

Chapter VI
The Massive Chest and How to Build It

THE muscles that contribute to the girth of the chest, as mentioned before, are the latissimus dorsi muscles of the back. For when this muscle is contracted, the chest measurement can be increased a great many inches. Nevertheless, attention should be paid to the pectoral muscles, which cover the upper part of the chest, as well-rounded and thick pectorals are rare even in splendidly developed athletes. Every devotee to physical culture has well-developed pectoral muscles, but very few have all the contour and thickness that can be obtained by scientifically applied exercise to these muscles.

A great many people have the erroneous idea that the pectoral muscles constitute the major girth of the chest. This is a mistake. Thick pectorals, however, will increase the size of the chest a couple of inches. But the principal point in their development is to obtain the maximum strength and co-ordination in your development, and at the same time attain a striking appearance, characterized by the splendid contour of perfect pectoral development. Thick pectorals will add greatly to the height of your chest, and strong pectorals will come in mighty handy in the performance of feats of strength.

How Push-up Exercises Develop the Pectoral Muscles

The well-known push-up exercise from the floor, sometimes called the "floor dip," will bring out the pectorals to a splendid degree, as will dipping on the parallel bars, or between chairs. These exercises are about the best to be had for this purpose. Yet additional resistance must be applied as the student progresses, and eventually, as his muscles become stronger and stronger, the number of repetitions will increase, until eventually he will be compelled to perform one hundred or more repetitions in order to tire the muscles used.

The pectorals should be tired within twenty-five counts, if possible. If further repetitions are called into play, the exercise becomes too light and considerable energy is lost. The push-up from the floor will not affect the pectoral muscles as directly as will dipping on parallel bars, owing to the fact that in this exercise the body is lowered further down between parallel bars than in the case of pushing up from the floor.

If the student prefers floor dipping, I suggest that he elevate his feet on a chair or stool, and that he perform his dipping between two low boxes or stools, so as to enable his chest to be lowered as far downward as possible, until he feels a great strain placed upon the pectoral muscles. In performing push-ups, whether it be on the floor, or between chairs, you cannot develop the pectoral muscles without developing the triceps and abdominal muscles as well, for all these groups are brought into play.

Direct Pectoral Exercise

If the student is desirous of putting direct application on the pectoral muscles, this can be done by clasping the hands in front of the chest and while resisting, pushing one hand as far as possible to the right, then pushing the other hand upon the return count as far as possible to the left, continuing this until both pectorals begin to ache.

I would not advise the student, however, to adhere strictly to this exercise, unless he is exceedingly deficient in pectoral development. For, as previously stated, when the muscles are exercised in groups, much better results can be obtained, as far as strength and co-ordination are concerned. When the student can perform more than twenty-five repetitions in a floor dip, or when dipping between chairs or bars, he should use some method of adding resistance. When exercising between the bars, he should utilize an adjustable weight tied to his feet. When the exercise is performed on the floor, he should use some elastic resistance, pulling against his body.

Having an adjustable weight with the loop arrangement, so as to loop it over the foot when dipping between the parallel bars, will compel you to lessen the repetitions and enable you to obtain all the strain you want, depending, of course, upon the amount of weight used.

The ambitious student can very easily secure elastic cables and manufacture a crude home-made harness to fit over his head or around the back of his neck, and with the cables attached to two screws on the floor, he can perform the push-up from the floor or between boxes, with the feet elevated on a chair, and thereby obtain much better results than if he performed the movement without any artificial resistance.

Of course, the use of a weight or elastic cables is not absolutely essential, as far as development is concerned, for the student will eventually obtain almost as good results by lifting the mere weight of his own body. However, it will take him longer to reach his maximum development.

Don't Neglect Your Light Exercises

Although I am an enthusiastic advocate of heavy work in physical culture, nevertheless, I am a firm believer in doing light exercises in conjunction with the heavy work, for if anyone does heavy work exclusively, he will eventually become slow in movement. Therefore, light work is essential, if you desire speed, combined with great strength and development.

You should not perform the light work, however, until you have first finished your drill with the heavy work, because light endurance work will consume your energy, and prevent you from the continuance of muscle-building exercise. You have just so much energy to expend at each drill, and no more. Therefore, when the point of fatigue is reached, it is the sign to stop. Light endurance work should be done as relaxation or play. Therefore, it is better to perform such work some other part of the day or evening, during your period of relaxation.

I suggest also that the student adopt handball, swimming, skating, tennis and similar competitive sports, in order to develop speed and endurance. Such pastimes, not being muscle-building work, will not develop you to any extent, so do not depend wholly upon these sports for benefiting your muscular system. They are of more benefit to your internal organs and lungs than anything else.

The student might also perform floor dipping without any artificial resistance, as a limbering-up exercise, to precede his muscle-building drill. In that case he would do well to continue the repetitions until the muscles begin to ache, whether these counts total twenty-five or one hundred and twenty-five, for this exercise, even though a strenuous one for the beginners, is really a very light one for the advanced pupil. Those who have not as yet reached their maximum degree of strength and development, will realize this as they progress. However, as stated for development, the student must arrange this floor-dipping exercise progressively and tire the muscles before the twenty-fifth count, otherwise it becomes a warming-up movement.

Don't Forget Your Deep Breathing Exercises

I am an enthusiast on deep breathing, and highly recommend the student to take at least ten or fifteen deep inhalations after each muscle-building exercise, while he is resting for the next movement, even though he may be considerably out of breath. Indeed, when you are out of breath, deep breathing is of special benefit.

Practice deep breathing at all times, whenever you think of it during the day, for you really cannot get too much fresh air in your lungs. Deep breathing is excellent for the expansion of the rib box and for stretching the cartilages of the ribs and sternum, thereby deepening and widening the chest. Several inches can be gained in chest measurement by increasing the lung capacity.

An individual with a narrow rib box cannot expect to acquire the depth and size of the chest of his wide rib boxed competitor. Nevertheless, deep breathing can change the shape of his rib box considerably. Inhale through the nose always, and always exhale through the mouth, when performing breathing exercises.

The lifting of a weight while lying on your back on the floor also benefits the pectoral muscles, but does not offer as complete a movement as dipping between parallel bars or chairs. Chinning the bar also brings into play the pectoral muscles to some extent, but not as strongly as dipping.

Building Health by Deep Breathing

One of the finest developed chests I ever saw, was built up largely through deep breathing exercises. This young fellow, only a few years before, had been advised to give up his work and go out on a ranch to live, for the doctor thought that he was far advanced in tuberculosis.

Circumstances were such with him at the time, however, that he could not possibly get away, as he would lose the result of several years' hard work in a little business he had built up in the East.

When he came to see me, and asked what I would suggest, under the circumstances, I told him that, to my mind, there wasn't any reason in the world why he couldn't develop his lung power, increase his health and his vital resistance, and maybe even overcome, to a very great extent, the ravages of his disease, and still remain in New York.

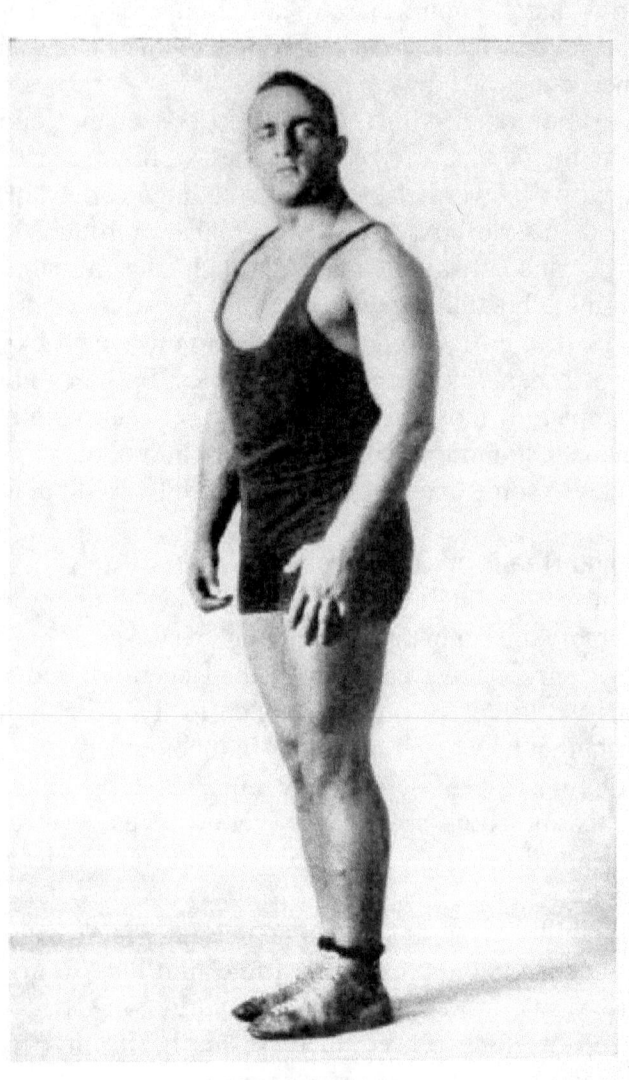

WLADEK ZBYSZKO
An interesting pose showing this splendid wrestler's remarkable depth of chest.

Under my instructions he started in to breathe properly. His progress was nothing short of remarkable. For, within three months he had gained two inches in lung expansion. I then put him on carefully selected exercises, calculated to develop his pectoral muscles and his lung capacity, and today, two years after he first came to me, he is entirely free from his tubercular condition. In fact, this same doctor now says: "He is the very picture of ruddy health." And he didn't have to go away or give up his business to get this, either, as he had been warned to do.

I don't tell you this for the purpose of creating any distrust in your doctor, or what your doctor tells you. I only tell you what any well qualified doctor will tell you; that is, that a good part of any cure of lung trouble must come from deep breathing exercises and the better nutrition which these exercises help to bring about.

You Can Enlarge Your Chest Four or Five Inches

Now, natural deep breathing will enlarge anyone's chest several inches in a remarkably short space of time. Yet you will find that nine people out of ten are actually too lazy to inhale to the fullest extent. In fact, the deepest inhalation of most cigarette smokers is when they inhale the poisonous smoke of cigarettes. If the reader will try and form the habit of taking at least fifty deep, long breaths every day, he will be amply paid for these efforts, not only in the increased size of his chest, but in the better supply of blood and increased vitality that he will gain from doing this. Continual deep inhalations expand the rib box, for every rib is joined together by cartilages, and these expand or contract with each inhalation. The sternum or breast bone also consists of cartilages, and this expands in unison.

In conjunction with the deep breathing, if you will apply systematic exercising to the pectoral muscles, which cover the upper chest, you can add another couple of inches to the size of your chest. If you will also apply systematic exercising to the latissimus dorsi muscle of the back, you will add many more inches to the size of the chest.

Don't Depend on Your Tailor for a Deep Chest

After reading this, how can anyone remain satisfied with a chest that is under-sized, and not up to the standard. With a deep, full chest, you won't have to depend upon the tailor to give you an athletic appearance. And you will also find that the increased blood supply in circulation, and the greater supply of oxygen, will give you the vitality and energy that only a well-trained athlete knows.

The pectoral muscles can be developed by numerous methods, but, after all, it is all based on one principle; that is, of cramping the muscles together, or contracting them. The student should be considerate and give more attention to the muscles of the back than to the pectoral muscles, for too much pectoral muscle has a tendency to bring the shoulders forward and give you a round-shouldered appearance. However, if the deltoid and back muscles are exercised in conjunction with the pectorals, no one need fear becoming round-shouldered.

A deep, full, well-developed chest is admired by all, and looks especially well under a top light when being photographed. Then, again, a good chest gives the owner a fine appearance when in bathing, especially when the sun is overhead, and deep shadows are cast under the pectoral muscles.

It is not uncommon for anyone who has practiced deep breathing and systematic chest exercises, including exercises for the muscles of the back, which help to increase the size of the chest, to have an expansion of over a foot. I myself can show a difference of 14 inches between contraction and expansion, and I have seen and measured a professional strong man whose expansion was over 18 inches. In fact, it is not at all uncommon for a well- trained athlete to be able to place a cup and saucer on top of his expanded chest, without it falling off.

Of Course, the Big-boned Man Again Has the Advantage

The big-boned man naturally has the advantage again over his small-boned neighbor. For the small-framed individual cannot and must not expect as broad a chest as one who possesses a wide, bony structure, and who has exceptionally wide shoulders. However, the small-boned athlete can develop a chest that he can be proud of, for he can increase his pectoral muscles to a thickness of several inches, and then undoubtedly have more depth to his chest than his broad-boned competitor. The broad- boned man, however, can have a much wider and broader chest, if he trains for it, and, of course, could attain much larger measurements.

There is another set of very pleasant-looking muscles of the chest called the serratus magnus, which consists of nine fleshy digitations, of which only five can be seen. These muscles are located on each side of the rib box.

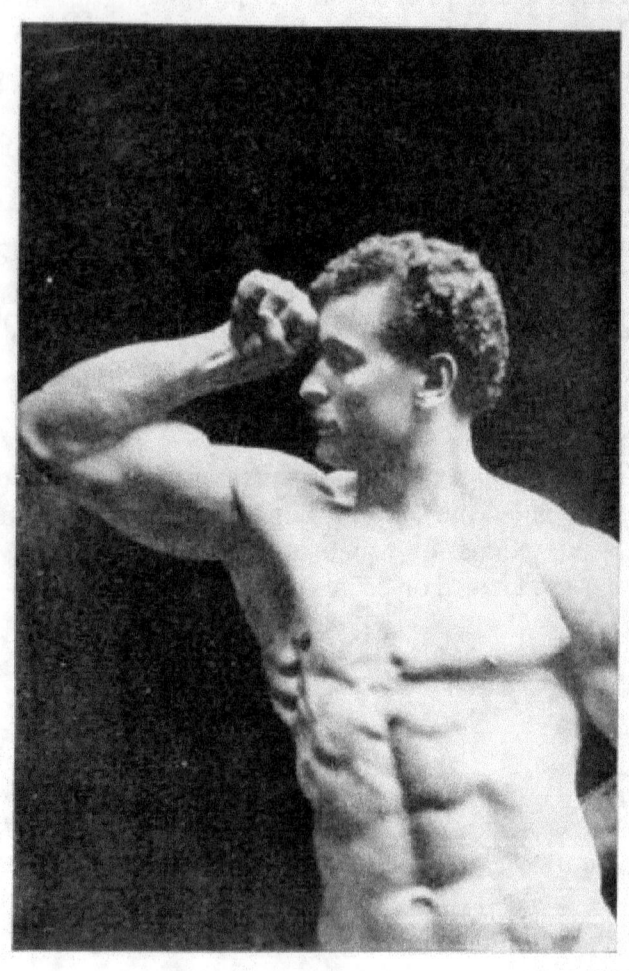

EUGEN SANDOW
An interesting display of the torso

How to Find the True Lung Expansion

To find the true lung expansion the measurement should be taken at the ninth rib. Then the student will find, much to his surprise, that he will not be able to expand more than one to three inches, depending upon the size of his rib box. The rib box must be taken into consideration in estimating chest development. Some people are fortunate in possessing ribs that are wide appearing in the front, while others have a frame-work that shows the ribs almost parallel with each other.

A person whose ribs are far apart generally has more endurance, more reserve energy and greater lung capacity than the person whose ribs are narrow. However, everyone's rib box can be enlarged, as I have stated. If you are not among the fortunate ones, there is no reason why you should not improve yourself to your limit and become stronger, more energetic and better developed than the average calisthenic student.

It was only a few years ago that a thin, sickly, flat-chested young man called on me. I examined him. He stood before me, and I carefully noticed his numerous defects. He had a narrow rib box, a rather deep hollow in the center of his chest. His back protruded from his round shoulders in a way that, if the same curve had been in front of him, would have given him a very high chest. If I recall rightly, his chest measured normal, about 32 inches. The other parts of his body were in no better proportion. He weighed about 115 pounds and was of average height.

For the first three months, all I had him do was systematic deep breathing—nothing else. No exercise in any form, except walking. After that I slowly progressed him with scientific exercises. Before one year was up, this chap had an all-around development and a chest that was his most prominent feature. He told me his friends called him "Chesty." This man continued progressive exercising and deep breathing, and after three years, has become one of the finest developed athletes America has ever produced.

His arms and shoulders and chest reached massive dimensions in spite of his small rib box. His legs have rounded out into wonderful proportions, while his strength has become more than six times greater than it was the day I first met him. I am simply quoting this as an example, to show what anyone can do if he so desires.

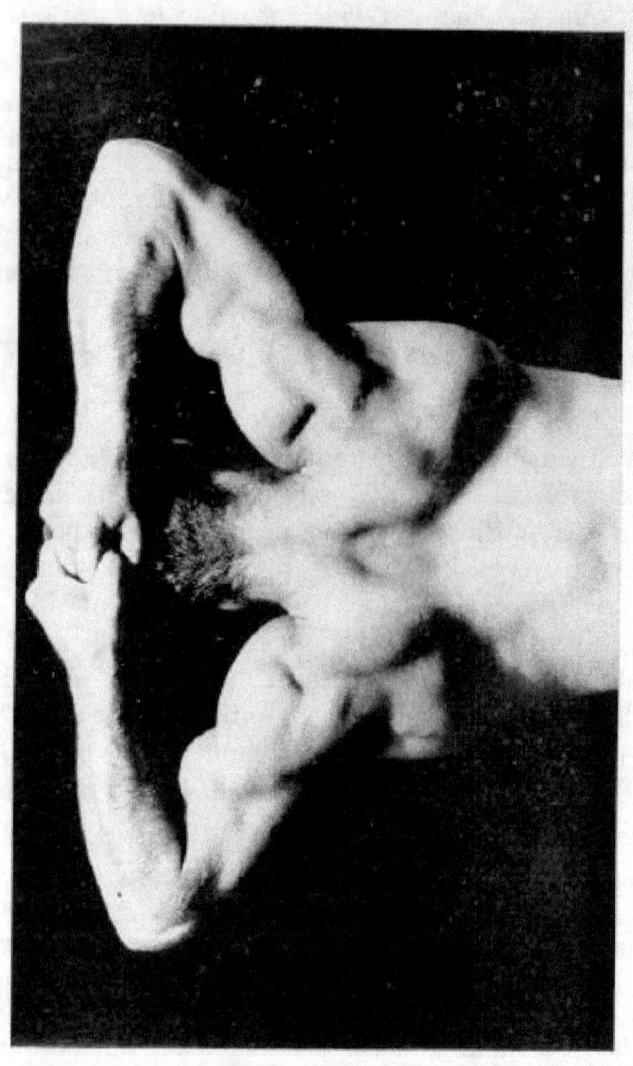

ARTHUR L. HYSON

The back development of this athlete is indeed remarkable. The formation of his back muscles change completely with the mere pressure and relaxation of his hands when placed upon his head.

So there is no need for anyone to continue to own a chest that he is not satisfied with. It is only a matter of making up your mind to build it up, and then "going to it."

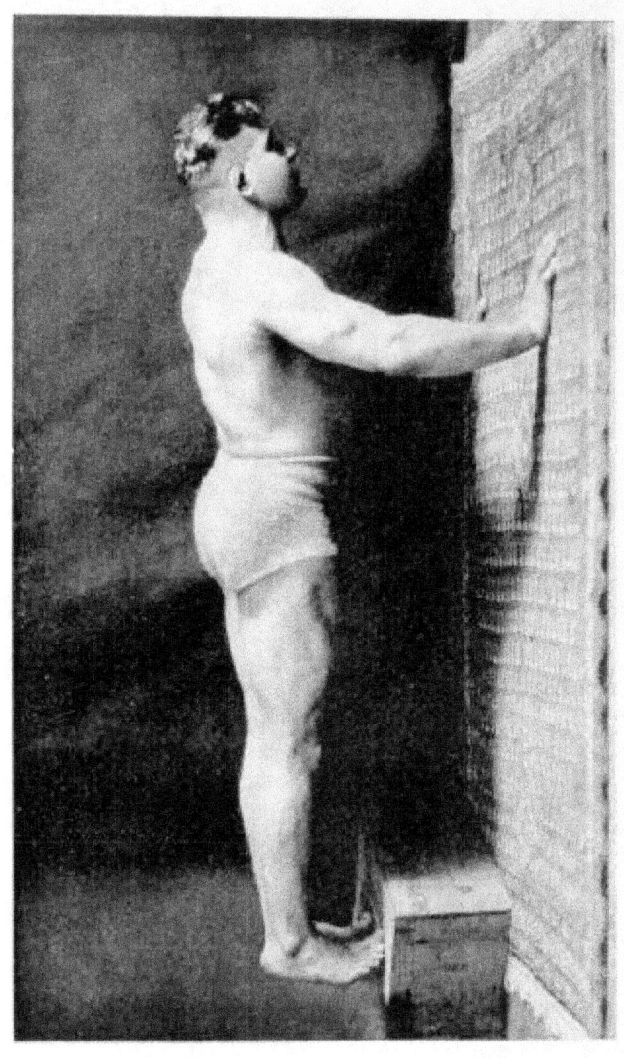

EXERCISE FOR THE CHEST AND ARMS

Push up and down from the floor, keeping the body stiff. This exercise can be made more difficult by elevating the feet as shown in the above photograph. (See chapter on the chest.)

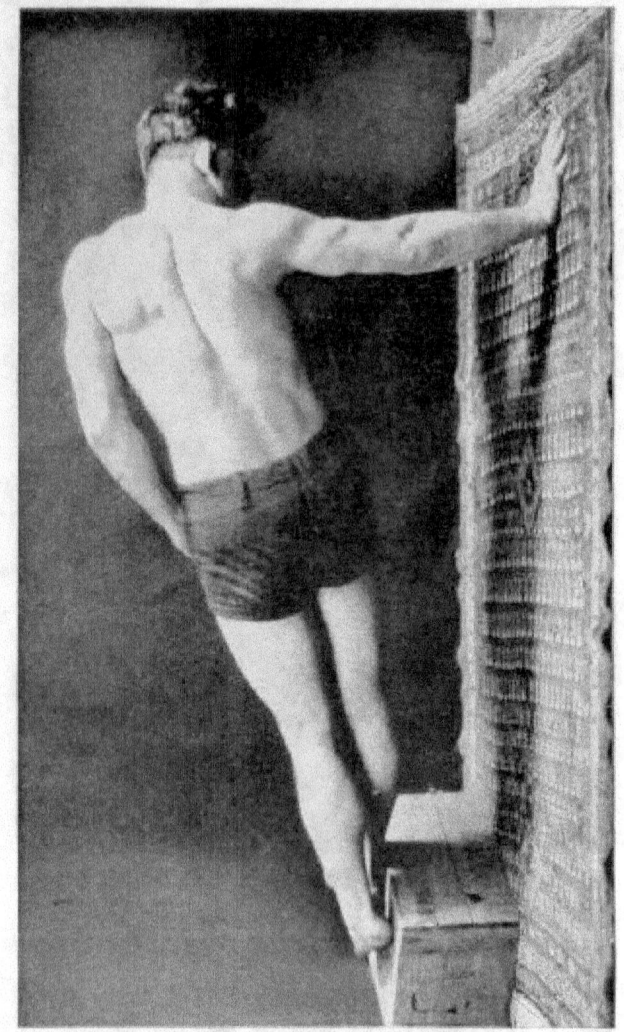

EXERCISE FOR THE CHEST AND ARMS

Pushing up and down from the floor on one arm at a time is quite
difficult and considerable strain is placed upon the triceps and deltoid
muscles. Yet it brings into play the pectoral muscle and is an excellent
means of broadening and deepening the chest. (See chapter on the
chest.)

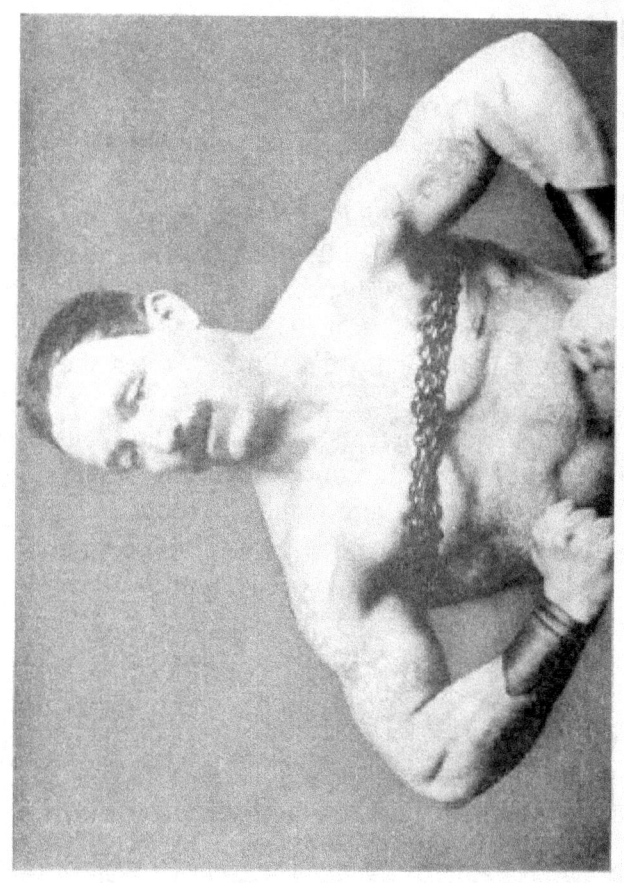

PIERRE GASNIER

*The circus strong man of the past generation whose performances en-
thused the author as a boy to strive for strength and development.*

Chapter VII
Splendid Arms and How to Have Them

FROM the early schoolboy days, the arms seem to be one part of the body in which everyone takes pride. As a boy we all can recall the enthusiasm with which we rolled up our sleeves to show the lump on our upper arm. When I was a boy, the one who had the biggest biceps was the boy to command the greatest respect. No thought was given to any other muscle of the arm, but the whole attention was centered on the little lump that formed when the fist was brought to the shoulder.

I also recall what interest and admiration was aroused in me when I went to the circus and saw the strong man there break chains that were wrapped around his arms. My admiration was not tampered with, but I discovered, in later years, that the chains had been tampered with. How discouraged I felt upon my return home when I beheld my own skinny arms in the mirror. The pair of arms that I then owned, measured but 9½ inches. I remember later how envious I was of a husky chap, while attending high school, whose arm measured, when flexed, 14 inches. My own arm measured about 12½ inches then. I think, however, that by envying as I did, it had considerable effect upon my progress, for it made me work harder to reach my goal. And it wasn't very many years before the arms that I had envied were soon much smaller and less developed than my own.

I realized then that the biceps was only one of the muscles in the arm, and that by proper application of exercises, the girth of my arms could be increased rapidly. I learned that the triceps, the muscles behind or underneath the arms, constituted the bigger bulk of the upper arms and, therefore, realized that special attention must be paid to these muscles. The average individual (unless he is a thorough student of anatomy and physical culture) sadly neglects the triceps, which, when properly developed, give a pleasing curve to the back of the arms, and also lend fullness to the size of the upper arms. These muscles are developed by constant pushing, whether it be downward, sideways or upwards. You must push against a strong resistance of some kind in order to develop these muscles to their maximum.

The Triceps Is Perhaps the Most Important Muscle in the Upper Arm

The reason I am beginning this chapter on the arms with the triceps muscle is that this is the strongest and largest and the most important muscle of the upper arm. It is called triceps because it has three heads. Its origin is from the border of the scapula or shoulder blade to the posterior or back surface of the humerus bone of the upper arm. Its insertion is in the olecranon process of the ulna, one of the two bones in the forearm.

Although the origin and insertion of the muscles are the same in everyone, still the triceps differ in appearance, just as much as other muscles are differently developed in various individuals.

The variations in appearance of this muscle depend somewhat upon the size of the bones, in the first place, and then again, upon the different exercises that each student uses toward development. Some people have what might be termed a "flat" triceps, while others have a "round" triceps. The difference is that a "flat" triceps has the internal head more highly developed than the external head, thereby giving the arm a wide appearance and great fullness in the back, when viewed from the side. When the external head is more highly developed than the internal head, the arm will not look as wide when viewed from the side, but it will look thicker when viewed from the front or from the back.

It is very difficult to set a standard as to the proper degrees of development of the internal head and of the external head, but in my opinion, considerable attention should be paid to both heads of this muscle, for when both are highly developed the arm will have width as well as thickness.

When the hands are placed upon the hips, you will undoubtedly notice in many athletes and strong men the curve on the top of the upper arm will vary in appearance. Some athletes have a very pronounced curve, while in others, the arm is smoother. This is caused by the different degrees of the external head of the triceps development.

I have also noticed in a number of cases, the triceps development varies greatly where the internal head breaks or protrudes up on the arm. I have seen remarkably developed athletes whose internal head of the triceps when flexed began slightly above the back of the elbow and gradually slanted outwards, until it reached its bulk about midway on the upper arm. Then I have seen equally well developed athletes whose triceps were practically straight from the back of the elbow until they reached the middle of the upper arm. Then the internal head gave a sudden break, or raise, until the muscle knotted up to its bulk a little above the middle of the upper arm.

Judging from the ability and strength of these two different types of athletes, I have found that when the triceps does not make so abrupt a break, but when the internal head extends downward with a pleasing slant toward the back of the elbow, the man has much more strength and endurance than when the internal head breaks sharply above the middle of the upper arm. Weight lifters, gymnasts, and apparatus workers, as a rule, have the internal head of the triceps longer than those who have developed this muscle by individual arm work.

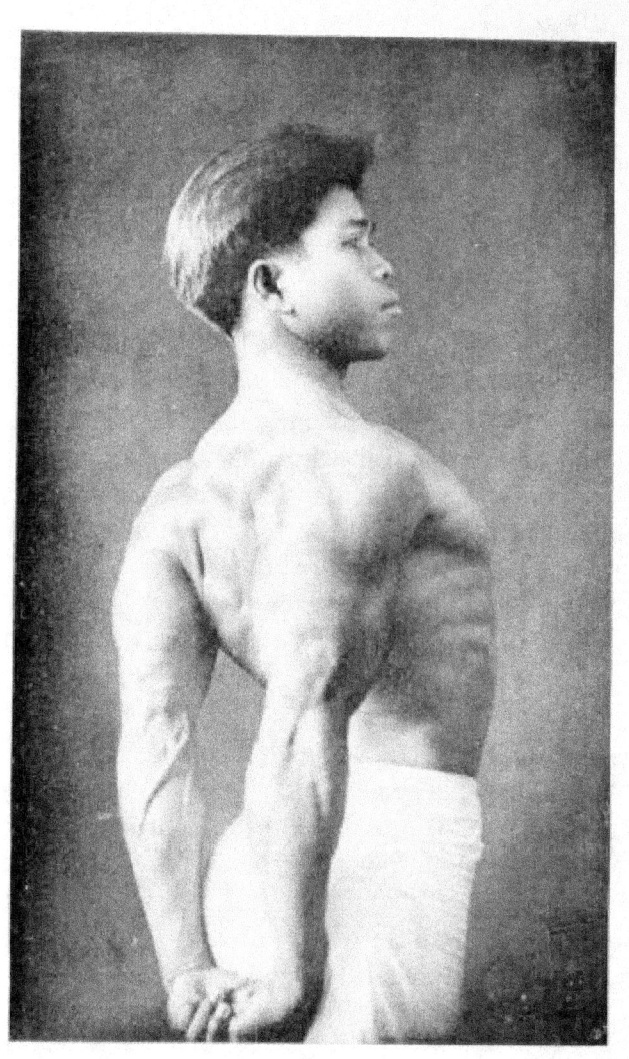

SIMON JAVILITO

This Philippine athlete possesses an exceptional arm development and an interesting view of the triceps can be had in the above pose.

Therefore, it can readily be seen that it is to the best advantage of the student to work the muscles in groups, if he desires not only co-ordination, but strength as well. Tensing or resisting exercises are excellent for bringing out the internal heads of the triceps muscle. But if the muscle is developed purely by such methods, it will be good for boxing or display, but for nothing else, and when put to a test in any kind of competition for strength, it will be found wanting.

When the internal head of the triceps is well developed, and when the arm is held at the height of the shoulder and stretched sideways, a full, pleasing curve will be seen underneath the arm. The greater the internal triceps development, the rounder the muscle appears. If the student possesses muscles that are supple, by the slightest quiver of his hand and forearm he can cause the triceps to move back and forth while holding the arm in this position, for when the triceps muscle is relaxed, it should be exceedingly soft.

The external head of the triceps is developed by pushing, especially in performing overhead work, such as lifting a dumb-bell one hand overhead, or pushing the hand overhead, while working against some artificial resistance. It also can be brought out to a marked degree by assisting the deltoid in raising the arm sideways, while working against a strong resistance. Hand balancing also is of great value to this external head.

A highly developed external head of the triceps muscle will show a pronounced cord running from the external head downwards in the middle of the arm, towards the supinator longus muscle of the forearm. This part of the triceps can only be seen in highly developed arms, and arms where all superfluous flesh is lacking.

I am obliged to call the reader's attention to Simon Javierto, who is undoubtedly a remarkable example of development in this muscle. The picture of his arm held straight will give you an idea of perfect triceps development.

George Hackenschmidt's Triceps

One of the largest triceps muscles I have ever seen, or felt, for that matter, was owned by George Hackenschmidt, formerly the world's champion wrestler. The internal head of his triceps was more powerfully developed than the external head, while the break or slant of the internal head of his triceps was over two inches in length. When taking into consideration the size of his upper arm when flexed, over 19 inches, there is little wonder at his remarkable triceps.

Hand balancers almost always have triceps development equaled, that is, both heads of this muscle are harmoniously developed. If you will notice the back of their arms the next time you attend one of their performances, you will have a better conception of this important upper arm muscle.

The muscle in front of the upper arm is a two-headed muscle, called the biceps. This muscle arises from a tuberosity of the scapula or shoulder blade and is inserted in the upper part of the radius bone of the forearm. The development in this muscle differs in various athletes. Sometimes the muscle has a long appearance, even when flexed, and in other cases, it has an egg-like appearance. Even though the biceps is the best-known muscle in the body, it very seldom attains its maximum development unless the student devotes special attention to its use. The length of the arm and the size of the bones also affect the appearance of this muscle, as they do other parts of the body. Nevertheless, the pupil can attain biceps that are not only huge in appearance, but strong as well.

How to Develop the Biceps

Any sort of curling exercise will develop the biceps, as also will chinning, rope-climbing, etc. The biceps should be exercised not only individually, but in coordination with other parts of the body as well, for if the student devotes individual attention to the biceps, to the exclusion of other muscles throughout the same exercise, his biceps will knot up, but they will not be of a strong character.

Most gymnasts, weight lifters, and apparatus workers have very strong biceps, owing to the nature of the work they do, although the biceps development in many of these cases is not up to the standard. This simply shows that special attention must be devoted to this muscle, if the student desires bulk and height to the muscle.

The biceps muscle varies considerably in formation on different individuals, as you no doubt have noticed when bathing or in gym work with other men, or even among your office or shop mates. Some men have a knotted, egg-shaped muscle, others have a knotted and exceedingly high biceps, which has a pointed effect at the top or belly, while others have biceps that do not knot up, but are much longer in appearance.

Long biceps undoubtedly have better contour when the arm is relaxed, but they are not as strong as biceps that knot up into a huge pointed lump on the belly of this muscle. There is also another shape to the biceps muscle which, on a large, heavily-muscled arm has the appearance of a baseball, that is, round from every point of view. This kind of a biceps muscle is much thicker as a rule than the pointed and long biceps, and is generally much stronger. Such formation can be seen on weight lifters, ring artists, etc. The biceps that knot up in egg-shaped appearance usually are best for posing purposes and for muscular display.

I have often noticed a common fault with the biceps among athletes. In a number of cases the lower head breaks or ends too soon, and does not extend as far downward toward the bend in the elbow as it should. This is caused by developing the belly of the biceps to a higher degree than the upper or lower parts of this muscle. Great care should be taken in exercising the biceps by starting the movement with the arm absolutely straight and stiff. The arm should then be brought upward toward the shoulder, as high as it will go. If the student neglects the complete contractions and extensions of this muscle, and stops the movement before the arm is straightened, he will develop the belly of the muscle to a greater degree, and also shorten the break in the lower part of the biceps. This, unfortunately, will give him a muscle that is not only inferior in appearance, but which will also be lacking considerably in competitive strength work.

Another example of how this can be brought about is shown in the common chinning exercise. You hang from the bar with the hands and endeavor to pull yourself upward, until your chin touches the bar. While performing this exercise, if you do not lower yourself until your arms are absolutely straight each time, you will shorten the biceps muscle.

A very common fault among beginners, especially those who start their physical career with light three-or five-pound dumb-bell exercises, is to never make a com- plete extension while performing biceps work, especially when the dumb-bells are held in front of them. In my opinion, complete extensions and contractions are of more importance than the number of repetitions. However, I will take this up later, in another chapter.

You should attach just as much importance to complete extensions of the triceps muscles as you do to the biceps muscles, in order to secure the best results. If the student neglects this, he will fail to develop either the internal or the external head of the triceps as thoroughly as he would if he extended his arm to his limit while performing each exercise.

Whether you are dipping on the floor or lifting weights overhead, or pushing an object away from you, you are doing it for exercise and development. Therefore, make sure the arm is straightened to its limit during each count.

You Can't Pay Too Much Attention to the Upper Arm

It is almost impossible for you to pay too much attention to the upper arms, for it is practically impossible to exercise or move the upper arms without working the shoulder, chest or back muscles. In my idea of standard development, it is hardly possible for an athlete to over-develop his arms. You see so many highly developed athletes whose legs are splendid and whose torso is remarkable, yet they lack the professional finish to their development, owing to the fact that their arms are one or two inches too small, in proportion to their other muscles. This can be clearly shown to the student of anatomy, if you observe carefully the various kinds of physiques on the bathing beaches or in gymnasiums. You very seldom see a professional boxer whose arms are proportionately developed, in harmony with his body; whereas wrestlers, as a rule, possess arms that are fairly well in proportion, although in most cases the arms are not as highly developed as they could be. Weight lifters as a rule, have large arms. I am convinced that anyone can secure arms in proportion to his other muscles if he will only work to develop them.

It is not necessary to become a wrestler. It is not even necessary to become a weight lifter as long as the student will exercise scientifically and work against a strong resistance, whether it be the weight of his body, or some artificial appliance. The main factor about arm development is that the student must do progressive work. He must increase the resistance more and more as his arms become larger and stronger, otherwise he will simply stand still.

How You Can Acquire a Big Arm

It is an easy matter to acquire a 14-inch flexed upper arm. It is quite difficult for the average-sized man to reach 15 inches, and it is even more difficult for him to attain 16 inches. However, inasmuch as small-boned men have exceeded 16-inch upper arms, time and time again, it shows it can be done. The writer has proof of this, not only upon his own person, but upon thousands of others whom he has trained, and who have reached their maximum proportions.

When attempting arm development, it is folly for anyone to perform endless repetitions of movements, if he desires muscular tissue. For continuous light movements, though they will give the pupil endurance, will never get him anywhere, as far as bulk and strength are concerned. The arms, in my opinion, should be tired in less than fifteen repetitions. If anyone can perform an exercise more than fifteen times, that exercise is too light for him. He should immediately adopt heavier progressive work.

It is essential, therefore, that the student employ artificial means for further arm development. Even in the ordinary chinning and dipping exercises, if the student can perform these more than fifteen counts, he must tie, or pick up weights with his feet, or else have an adjustable elastic resistance that could be more and more progressive, if he expects to reach the maximum in the muscles he is using.

Vigorous attention to the biceps not only hardens them, but it brings a greater supply of blood to this muscle, thereby causing it to swell upon completion of the exercise. The student will soon learn that by swelling the muscles up to their maximum size within fifteen counts he will accomplish better results than by working against a resistance light enough for a school boy.

It is this constant swelling up of the muscles that increases their size. Therefore, if the pupil will give his triceps and biceps vigorous work, tiring both of them thoroughly, until they are fairly aching, he will discover his arms will be from ¼ to ½ inch larger when flexed than they were before, depending greatly, of course, upon his development.

Would You Like to Gain an Inch Next Month ?

The student who is desirous of gaining an inch around his upper arm during the next month will find that this is not difficult by scientifically applied exercise to his biceps and triceps. All he need do is to exercise these muscles sufficiently every day to swell them to their limit. If the arm swells up ½ inch after exercising, it does not stay that way the rest of the day, but diminishes at least 15/32 of an inch, retaining 1/32 as an increase.

The first two weeks the student will undoubtedly gain of an inch, whereas the next two weeks he should not expect to gain more than ¼ of an inch. The pupil will find that he will make more progress the first six months of the year than he will the last six months. For as the muscles become hardened and more developed, he will find it more and more difficult to increase their size. This simply verifies what I said before, that it is not so easy to attain a 16-inch arm. It means patience and hard work. In weight lifting, a pupil can very easily in a very short space of time and without any previous experience, lift 100 pounds overhead with two hands, but he cannot expect to lift 200 pounds with two hands during the next equal period. If he lifts 125 pounds he will be very fortunate. The same thing applies to the muscles.

A beginner who has never had any experience with training at all, and whose arm measures, for example, 12 inches when flexed, can attain, within three months, a 13½-inch arm. During the next three months his arm will measure 14 to 14½ inches. But during the next six months he will be very fortunate if his arm increases to 15 inches in size. The larger the upper arm becomes, the shorter it appears. Therefore, an athlete whose upper arm measures 17 to 17½ inches, providing he is of average height, generally gives the impression that his arms are short, when, in reality, his reach is just as long as it was when he started. This, as a rule, equals the height.

Don't Expect to Develop Large Biceps from Ordinary Calistlienic Work

A student of average height who endeavors to develop his arms by light calisthenic work, can never expect to attain more than a 14½-inch upper arm when flexed. Whereas the student who adopts progressive work, making the resistance stronger and stronger as he progresses, will not only save considerable time and energy, but he will develop muscles that are both huge in appearance and will be equal to any test of strength.

The individual with large bones again has the advantage over his small-boned competitor. A large-boned man develops upper arms that are not only stronger than his small-boned competitor, but arms that are more massive in appearance. On the other hand, the small- boned man may develop much finer looking arms, arms more suitable for photographing, owing to his small joints, than a large-boned man.

The small-boned individual, however, should not feel discouraged, for a 16-inch upper arm on a small-boned man looks much larger than a 17-inch arm on a big- boned individual, assuming, of course, that the individual has reached his maximum development.

Size of the arm counts but little if the development is not there, and many fleshy people who have large arms do not present the appearance of a thinner type individual whose arms are well trained. I have noticed in a number of cases that a well-developed 14-inch or 14½-inch upper arm looks a great deal larger than a 15½-inch upper arm, if the larger arm is not fully developed, even though both individuals are of the same height.

The forearm has considerable to do with the appearance of the upper arm, especially if the supinator longus muscle is thoroughly developed. The supinator longus muscles covering the upper and outer part of the forearm, pleasingly blend with the biceps, and if the pronator muscles on the inside of the forearm are roundlv developed, it will set off the upper arm considerably.

Don't Neglect Your Forearm If You Want Symmetry

It is a difficult thing to develop the upper arm without developing the forearm, although if the student desires exceptionally developed forearms, he must devote special attention to them. I have seen athletes who are an exception to this rule. One strong man, in particular, whom I know, has remarkable upper arms, measuring over 16 inches, whereas his forearm measured less than 12 inches. There is a reverse to this. I have seen athletes with remarkable forearms whose upper arms seemed small in comparison, although they were above average measurement. This is commonly noticed on individuals whose bones are unusually large. The small-boned man, as a rule, has small forearms, thereby exaggerating his upper arms and making them look even larger than they really are.

It is exceedingly difficult to set a standard for the forearm and the upper arm development as to ideal measurements, but my idea as to pleasing proportions is a 16-inch upper arm and a 12½-inch forearm; the forearm measurement, of course, being taken with arms straight. In order to find out the largest measurement of the forearm, the arm should be almost fully bent at the elbow, the fist clenched and the wrist turned down, and the tape passed around the largest part. A well-developed forearm will show a difference of from two to three inches from a relaxed to a flexed state in this manner. A well-developed forearm looks even more developed when the muscles of the wrist are pronounced. The student will find that the muscles above the wrist will increase the measurement of the wrist slightly when thoroughly developed, especially the extensor muscle which covers it.

Bending and turning the wrist, either with a weight or against a strong resistance, is undoubtedly the best possible means for the development of the forearm. The repetitions of this group of muscles should not exceed fifteen or twenty counts. If the student can perform a greater number of repetitions than this, he should increase the weight or resistance, so as to bring about maximum development in the shortest possible time.

Exercising the Arms

Now, as I have just said—and I cannot too strongly emphasize this fact—you cannot expect to develop strength in your arms unless strength is used in the movements. Therefore, anyone who continues light repetitions will never develop his biceps and triceps to their maximum. The work should be progressive, that is, the resistance should be increased as the muscles become stronger, just as you should do with other parts of the body. I cannot repeat this too often.

You need not be afraid of straining the arms too severely, for no serious result can arise by performing too vigorous movements or too heavy movements with the arms. The biceps should be tired within ten counts. Any exercise you do that carries the repetitions beyond ten counts in order to tire the biceps is much too light for you, and you should therefore increase the resistance.

The act of bending or flexing the arm, that is, starting from a straight position and bringing the fist toward the shoulder, constitutes the best means of developing the biceps muscle. If you pay attention to complete extensions and contractions of each movement, the biceps will develop to its fullest extent. Then if you desire strength and additional bulk to this muscle, you must increase the resistance or weight, as you progress with the work.

The strength of the biceps muscle really depends upon the kind of work the individual performs. I have previously mentioned the various shapes and strength elements, based on my observation and experience in physical training.

Heavy weights are excellent for strengthening and developing the biceps, and if persistent progress is made, the student will very quickly notice increase in the size of this muscle.

If you want to progress, you cannot expect to use the same weight continually, and expect to gain strength in your biceps. Whether you utilize weights or some other apparatus, the resistance should be increased one or two pounds each week, and even more, according to your strength and progress.

The resistance should be so graded that the biceps begins to feel uncomfortable about the fifth or sixth count, and at the eighth count it should start to ache. The ninth count should be done with effort, the tenth count with all the strength your arm possesses, and you should not be able to perform the eleventh repetition.

If you can tire your biceps muscle in this sort of work in even eight repetitions, it will strengthen your muscle much quicker. However, from experience, I have found that about ten repetitions are the best. The first four or five counts do not benefit you, as far as strength and development are concerned, as the last four or five repetitions do. It is when your muscles begin to feel uncomfortable and you force them to do additional work that they develop and strengthen. This is the secret of the success of the strong man.

If you will accept my suggestions and advice in these matters, and put them into practical application—and then keep at it—you will develop in a way you never dreamed of, and be a source of wonder to all your friends, who will marvel at your progress.

Just Because You May Be a Physical Culture Enthusiast Is No Proof that You Are Well Developed

About ninety-five out of one hundred men and boys exercise in some form or other, yet out of these ninety- five physical culture enthusiasts you seldom find one well-developed individual. The reason for this is that ninety-four of them discontinue exercising a muscle as soon as a slight uncomfortable feeling is felt. Consequently the proper amount of work is never given the muscles. The ninety-fifth individual is the one who continues the repetitions and uses the proper amount of resistance, causing his muscles to ache, and thereby attaining the health, strength and development to which everyone aspires.

I would not advise this severe progressive work with any other part of the body except the arms and shoulders, for if too much strain is placed on other parts, serious results might ensue. Yet the student need not have any fear of working his arms too much, providing he is not exercising them in co-ordination with his remaining muscles of the body.

If you perform, for example, a two-armed curl with an exceedingly heavy bar-bell, you are, of course, giving the biceps vigorous work and tiring them within ten counts, but while you are straining them with this bar bell, you are also straining your abdominal muscles and various other muscles in your body as well, and remember, "a chain is no stronger than its weakest link." Some day something might snap. To avoid this, it is best to strengthen the arms individually during the first six months, if it is the arms you are particularly desirous of benefiting. And when working the arms individually no fear need be had of over-straining.

Don't Rupture Yourself Lifting a Bar-bell

As I have previously stated, I am a firm believer of exercising the muscles in groups. However, when performing group work and using the arms to co-ordinate with other muscles in your body, I advise the student to "watch his step," and experiment a month or two first with only medium heavy work, so as to strengthen the various other muscles brought into play when performing a two-arm curl with a bar-bell. This lack of preparation and development is the most serious objection I have to using heavy weights. The student is apt not to gauge his movements properly, and in consequence he may be handicapped for several years with a rupture. I have seen so many weight lifters ruptured that I shrink from advising the student to adopt weight lifting in his first endeavors to develop his physique. To avoid even the slightest possibility of any such result I advise the student to perform different methods of exercising for the first six months with an exerciser, the resistance of which will increase the further it is stretched.

The great advantage of an elastic exerciser is that at the beginning of the movement, there is absolutely no resistance whatever. However, the resistance increases as the arm begins to flex. Therefore, the more you flex your arm, the further you stretch the elastic and the greater you increase the resistance.

By having an adjustable exerciser of this character, you will be able to add additional cables as your strength increases, thereby making the work progress in accordance with your own progress. There is not so much tendency to develop a strain when the movement is half completed as there is in the beginning of a movement, and when the movement is wholly completed, there is hardly any danger at all of becoming strained.

An example of this can be shown with a two-arm curl of a heavy bar-bell. If the bar-bell should be too heavy for you, in fact, almost impossible for you to curl it, the effort you put forth in the endeavor will cause considerable strain around the abdominal region. If, however, you have managed to curl the bell so that the arms are a little more than half flexed, the strain will lessen, and when the curl is completed and the bell held firmly at the top of the chest, the only strain you will experience is practically the pressure of the weight on your hands.

If you use a bar-bell not very difficult to start on the curl, and which places very little strain upon your co-ordinated muscles, you will find the bell much lighter as your biceps flex. For the biceps when flexed are more capable of performing heavier work than they are at the beginning of their flexion.

Therefore, it is better, in my opinion, to begin a movement with an apparatus that offers very little resistance at the beginning of a curl, and the resistance of which increases considerably as you flex your arms, for, as I have stated before, the arms become much stronger when the biceps becomes flexed.

Flexed Biceps Strength

Another example of this can be shown in chinning the bar. It is comparatively easy for anyone who has exercised even to a slight degree to perform the ordinary two-hand chin; that is, to pull the weight of the body up until the chin is over the bar. However, it is a very difficult feat of strength for even a trained athlete to perform a one-hand chin. On the other hand, it is a simple matter for the beginner to chin himself with two hands and lean all the weight to one side, while his chin is over the bar, holding himself up with the strength of his one arm alone.

This simply shows the strength of the biceps muscle when it is thoroughly flexed, and goes to prove what I have been telling you. The fact that it is easy for anyone to hold himself at the completion of the chin with his chin over the bar with one hand, while he would find it impossible to begin to chin himself with one hand alone, shows that the strength of the biceps muscle at the start of the movement is greatly inferior to its strength at the completion of a movement.

Therefore, it can readily be seen that the beginner, up to a period of six months, should not attempt heavy weight lifting for developing purposes. If he has obtained a fairly good physique, I recommend the use of heavy bar-bells and weights for strength and development purposes, providing he does not let his enthusiasm overwhelm his efforts. For, in my opinion, it is much better to be on the safe side and perform exercises systematically, with some scientific apparatus, rather than be in a hurry to strengthen and develop his muscles and make himself liable to a serious strain or a possible rupture. The muscles can be tired more systematically within ten repetitions with the use of a progressive elastic apparatus than they can with the use of a heavy dumb-bell.

Suggestion for the Triceps

The triceps, or the muscles behind the upper arm, must be exercised just the reverse of the biceps; that is, the movements must be of pushing instead of pulling. Dipping between parallel bars is excellent exercise for this muscle, for it not only strengthens and develops the triceps, but it plays upon the pectorals and other muscles as well. As I suggested in the chapter on the chest, you should perform this dipping between parallel bars (or chairs, if you have no bars), with a weight or other resistance tied to the feet in order to make it progressive.

The beginner may find this dipping between parallel bars a bit too strenuous. In that case I suggest he perform dipping or push-up on the floor until the triceps and pectorals become strong enough to try it between parallel bars.

The use of a moderately heavy weight is also excellent for the triceps. The movement is started from the shoulders and extended to arm's length overhead. I would not advise the student to use a heavier weight than he is able to press up with a very slight bend at the opposite side of his waist, for if the weight is too heavy, he will have to resort to a bent-press movement. A bent- press exercise is entirely too severe for the beginner, and should only be indulged in after the student acquires a fair amount of strength and development and is desirous of testing for strength a few times a week.

If you are more enthusiastic about heavy weights than any other apparatus, I suggest you do not use them more than two or three times a week, for the use of weights oftener than this will have a tendency not only to slow you up, but it will tear down the tissues more quickly than they can be replenished. In order to acquire the best results from exercising with heavy weights, the work should be done about three times a week, thereby giving periods of rest in which to recuperate and build up the muscles.

In advocating heavy weights, understand, I am doing it merely for strength purposes, and not for development. For as I have said, far greater progress can be made in developing by other means of exercise. To the person who does not use heavy weights, I suggest he exercise daily, for exercising for development purposes is not as hard, or as straining as exercising for strength purposes, and consequently fifteen to thirty minutes daily spent on the physical welfare of your body is not too much time. Whereas, if the student followed the every-other-day program, as in weight lifting for strength purposes, it would not be sufficiently rapid progress for his development.

The triceps, being a three-headed muscle, is much stronger than the biceps, which has but two heads. Therefore, a greater amount of resistance can be applied to the triceps than to the biceps. If you are desirous of developing the triceps rapidly and to their maximum degree, you must not use the same weight or resistance that you use to exercise the biceps with, but you should increase this resistance at least 25 per cent, or more.

For example, if you are working with the biceps against a resistance of 50 pounds, you should add at least 12 to 15 pounds more, if you use the same weight or apparatus to exercise the triceps. This percentage will vary greatly with different people.

The average untrained person possesses biceps that are much stronger than his triceps, but after he has been exercising for a short while, his triceps soon excel his biceps in strength. It will, therefore, be possible to use a weight or resistance in exercising his triceps, that he will find impossible in exercising his biceps. For instance, the untrained individual can chin himself more times than he can dip, but after he has practiced both for a short period, he will be able to dip more times than he can chin.

Exercises for the Upper Arm

There are hundreds of various forms of exercise that can be used for strengthening and developing the upper arm. The few I recommend here I have found to produce results quickly:

EXERCISE 1. Stand erect. Hold bell at sides. Bring bell to shoulders. Thoroughly flex the arm and lower again until the arm is straightened. Repeat. This can be performed also with a progressive exerciser. At the same time use a heavy enough bell or strong enough resistance in the exerciser until the muscle is aching. This aching point should be reached within ten repetitions. I would not advise a beginner to use a bar-bell and both arms at the same time until he has obtained a considerable degree of strength and development, but the arms should be worked individually in this biceps exercise.

EXERCISE 2. Bend forward and lift the bell off the floor about two inches. Then curl bell to shoulders, without touching any part of the arm to the body. This works the biceps muscle, but in a much harder way, and will naturally tire the muscle quicker. The weight of the bell should be increased as the muscle strengthens. In no case have the bell so light that it will not tire your muscles out in ten repetitions if you desire to make rapid progress in the development of the biceps muscle.

Now do both of these exercises with a somewhat lighter weight, but begin the curl with the palms reversed, so that when the curl is completed, the palms will be facing the floor. This will work the biceps in a different way, and also call into play the supinator muscles of the forearm. You may find in this case that the supinator longus muscle of the forearm will tire before the biceps.

While exercising the arms you should concentrate your attention on the muscle used, for this will stimulate the effort and help you with your progress. If you allow your mind to wander when doing these exercises, or any exercise, in fact, you will not get as much good out of them as you would if you devoted your entire attention to this movement. Think about the muscles you are exercising and, if possible, stand in front of the mirror, to watch them work.

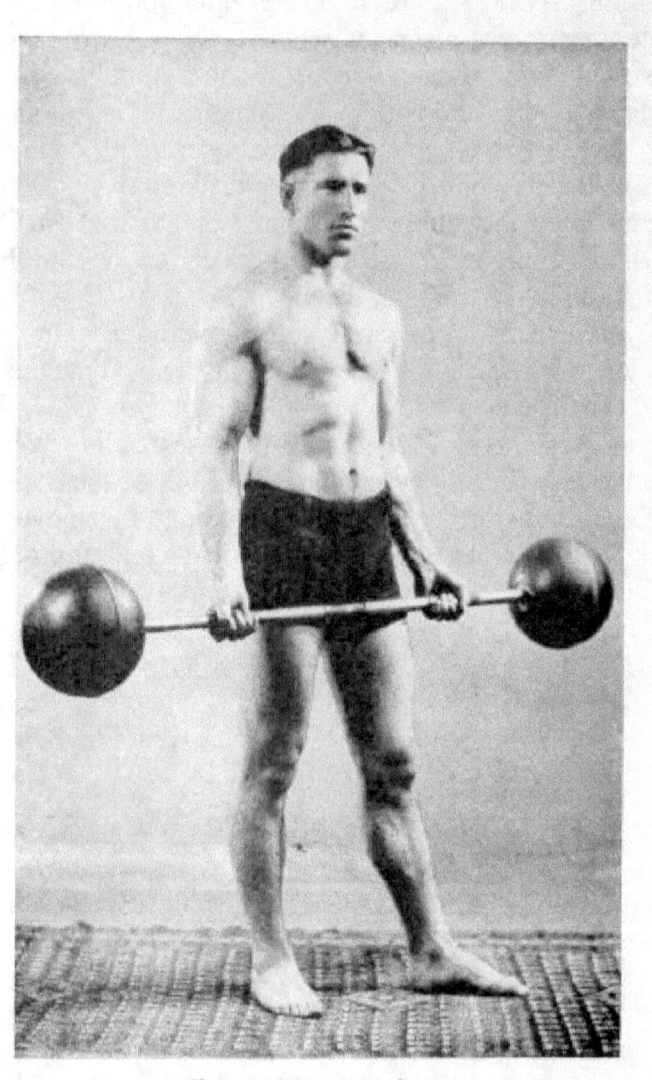

EXERCISE FOR THE ARMS

Hold barbell in front with arms stiff and palms forward.

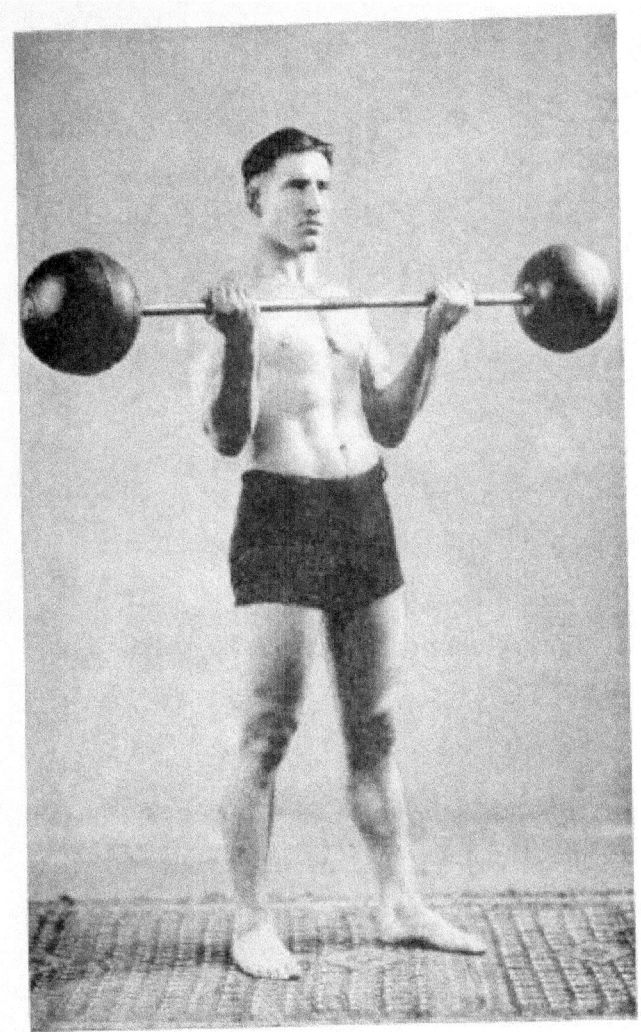

EXERCISE FOR THE ARMS

Then curl bell upwards by bending elbows, until bell is at height of shoulder and arms thoroughly flexed. For biceps muscle. (See chapter on the arms.)

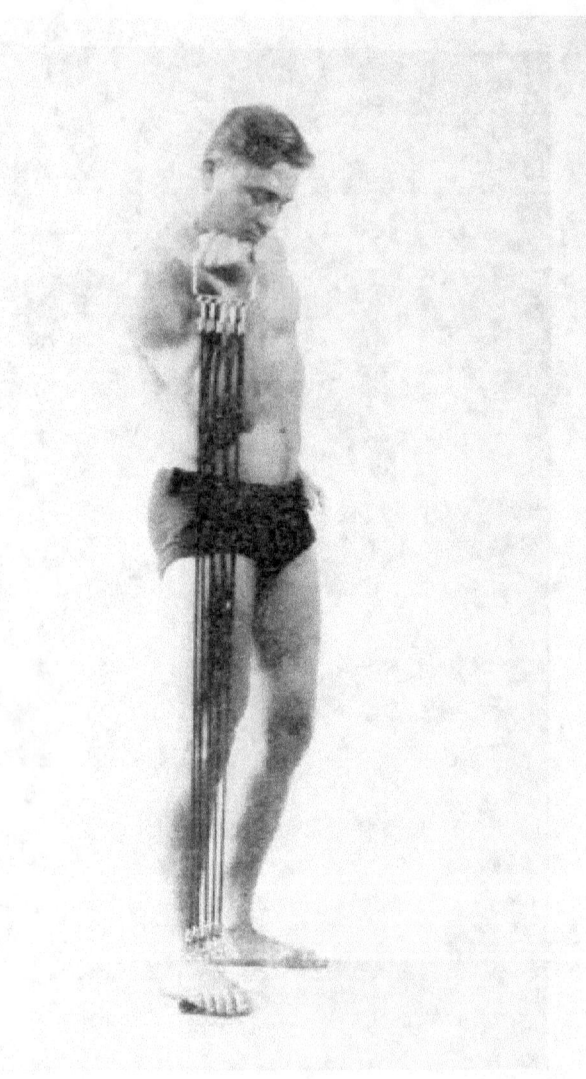

EXERCISE FOR THE ARMS

Another exercise for working the biceps muscle individually. Start movement with arms straight at side and then bend elbow by curling exerciser to height of shoulder as shown above. (See chapter on the arms.)

Chinning the Bar Is Good Exercise

Do plenty of chinning-the-bar exercises. If you can chin the bar more than ten counts, tie a weight to your feet. Whether you use a dumb-bell with a rope arrangement, or whether you make use of elastic cables for this purpose, you will find it will help your progress considerably in the development and strengthening of the biceps muscle.

If you are able to chin yourself with a 50-pound dumb-bell tied to your feet, you should make attempts at the "one-arm chin." This is a matter of practice. If you will endeavor to keep the palm of your hand and arm facing your body your efforts will be better in attempting this one-arm chin than if you allowed your body to turn while hanging by one arm before beginning this chin.

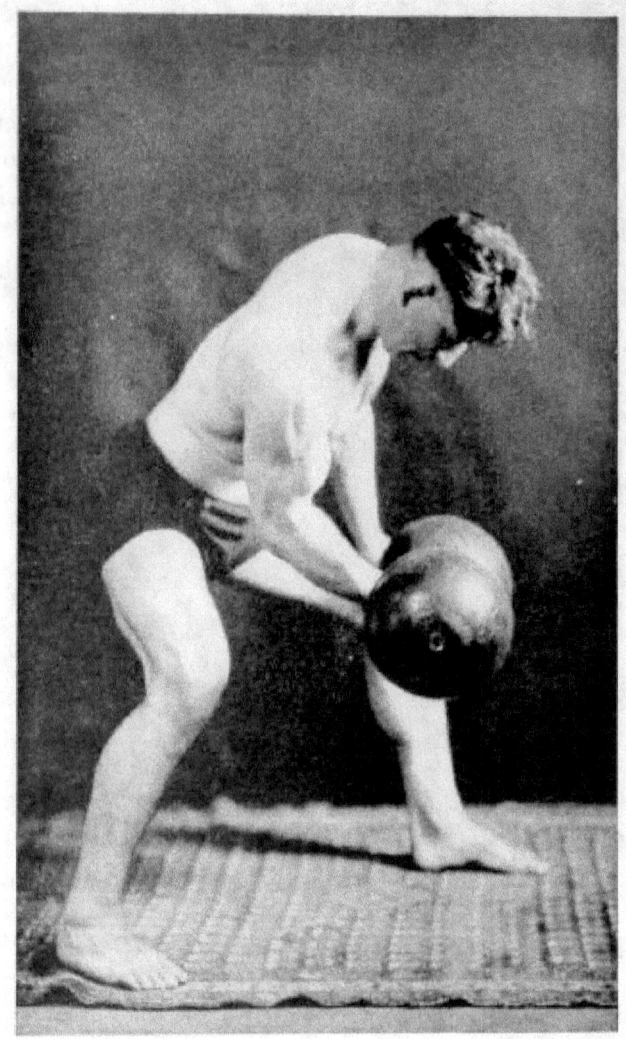

EXERCISE FOR THE ARMS

Curling a dumb-bell puts greater stress on the biceps than a bar-bell, and an advanced exercise is to flex arm without touching elbow to body, as shown above. Start with arm straight and bring bell to shoulder. (See chapter on the arms.)

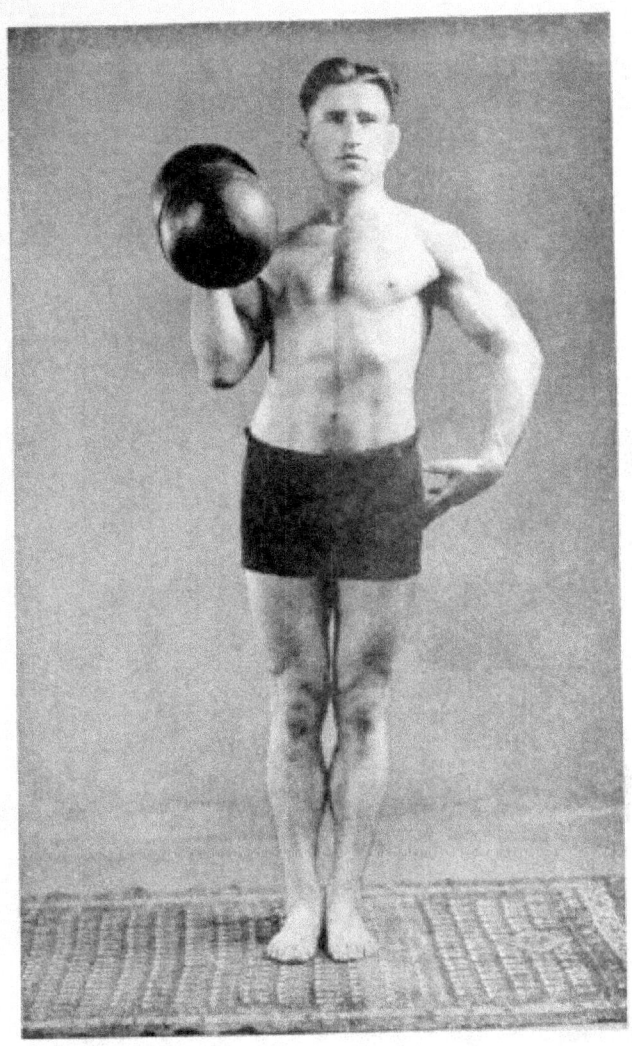

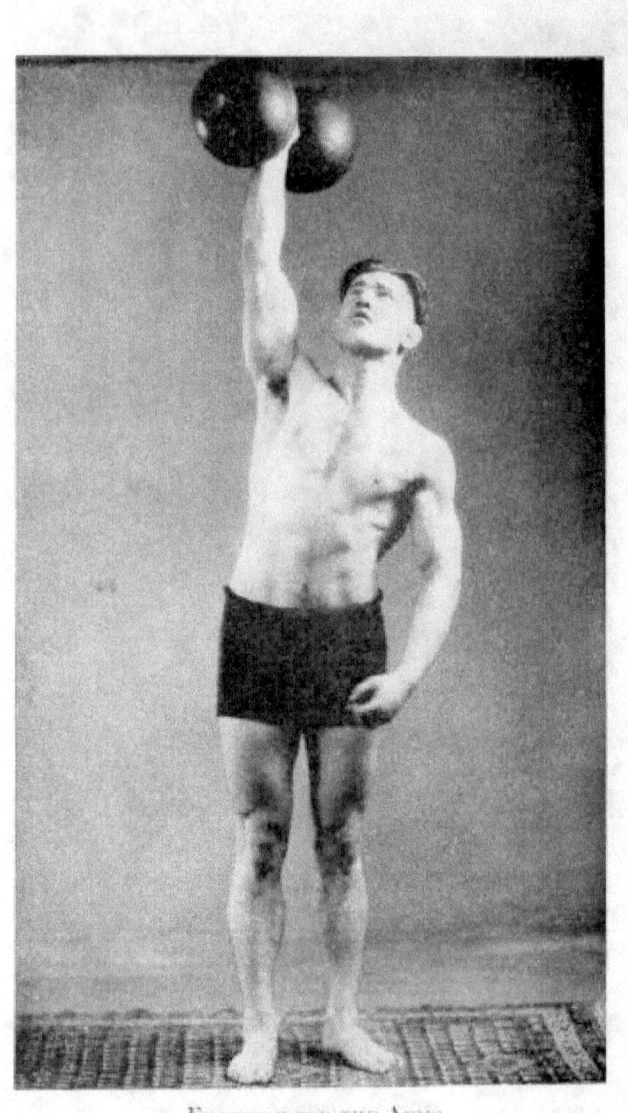

EXERCISE FOR THE ARMS

Stand erect with dumb-bell at height of shoulder.

EXERCISE 3. Hold the dumb-bell at the shoulder and push to arm's length overhead. This should be done in a military fashion. In other words, do not bend at the waist any more than you can help. If the weight should be so heavy that it compels you to bend sideways, be sure to keep the palm of your hand facing your body. Do not turn the wrist. The beginner may find his deltoid or shoulder muscle the first muscle to tire in this exercise, but with constant practice, he will strengthen his shoulder muscle so that the main resistance will apply to the triceps.

I find that excellent results can be accomplished in this exercise by the use of a progressive exerciser. If the exerciser is held behind the back with one arm still and the other arm ready to begin the movement at the height of the shoulder, as shown in the illustration, the triceps will receive more individual work in the upward push, because of the gradual increase of resistance as the exerciser is stretched. When the arm is at your shoulder, you have practically no tension or weight pressing on your hand with the use of this apparatus. But the further you push your hand overhead, the stronger the resistance becomes and the more your triceps muscle is put into play.

In performing arm work, always be sure to do the same amount of work with the left arm as you do with the right. Do not perform additional movements with your right arm because it may be stronger. If your left arm is weaker than the right, and is lacking in contour or development, you should endeavor to perform one or two extra counts on the left side, in order to eradicate all defects and develop your arms to symmetrical, equal proportions.

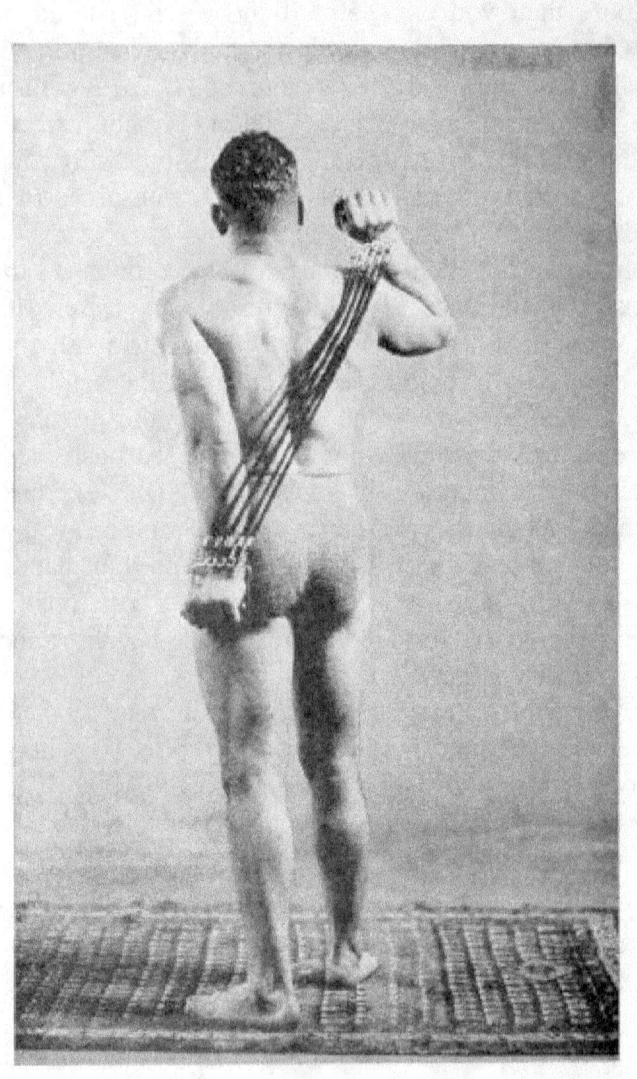

EXERCISE FOR THE ARMS

Another excellent exercise for the triceps can be had through the use of an exerciser. Hold expander behind back as shown above.

EXERCISE 4. Hold the exerciser over-head with one arm and have the other hand at the height of the corresponding shoulder. Then, while keeping the exerciser held aloft, with arms stiff, push other hand downward until the arm becomes straightened. This also gives the triceps plenty of work, and with the proper resistance, the muscle can be easily tired in less than ten repetitions.

EXERCISE 5. Hold bar-bell at height of the shoulder and with legs spread forward about 12 or 18 inches, press the bell slowly upward, until the arms are straight. Then lower, and repeat. Have the weight adjusted so as to tire your muscles within ten repetitions. This also affects the triceps directly, and will strengthen and develop them.

The reader must not confuse dumb-bell or bar-bell exercises with the term "heavy weight lifting for strength purposes." If the student does but the few bar-bell and dumb-bell exercises I have outlined, he can perform them daily, but if he attempts to see how much he can lift every day, or performs exercises so strenuous that he is unable to do more than three or four repetitions, he should not attempt this arduous work more often than three times a week. Otherwise he will become "stale" by not giving the muscles a chance to build up.

There is no need for me to give a list of exercises for the biceps and triceps here, because the reader can easily outline additional work for himself, if he so desires. I am simply outlining a few exercises for each muscle and the student can easily develop his entire body by performing the movements I have outlined for him in these pages.

I have also given the reader a choice between a barbell and a progressive exerciser, to adopt whichever he prefers, and according to his experience with training. If you are a beginner, take my advice and leave cumbersome bar-bells alone and use an elastic exerciser; but if you have over six months' experience with heavy work, then you need have no fear in attempting bar-bell work.

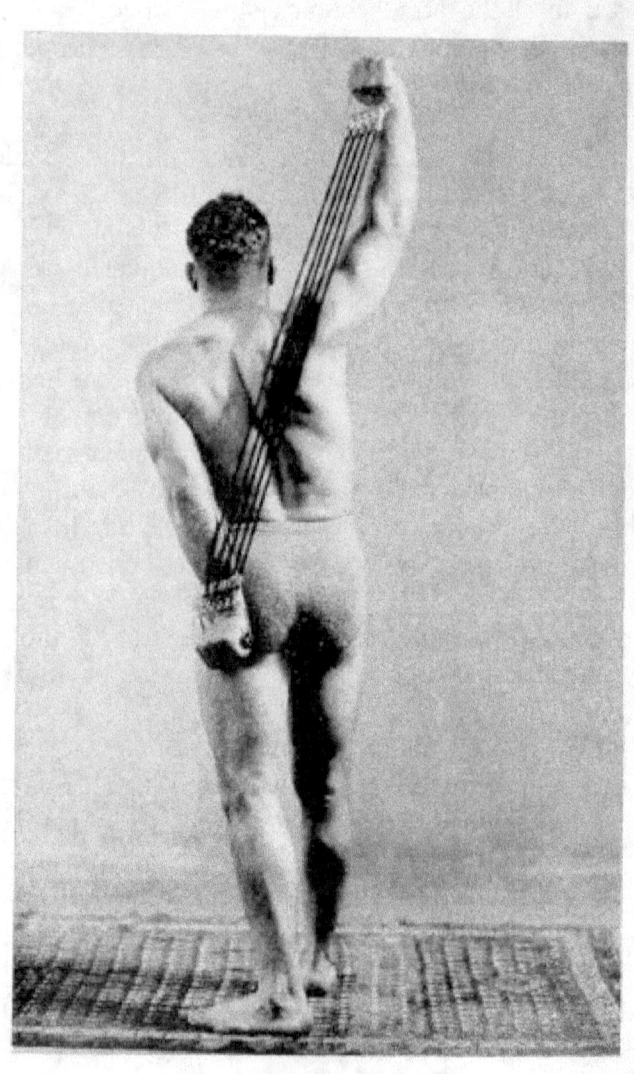

EXERCISE FOR THE ARMS

Then push arm upwards until arm is straight. (See chapter on arms.)

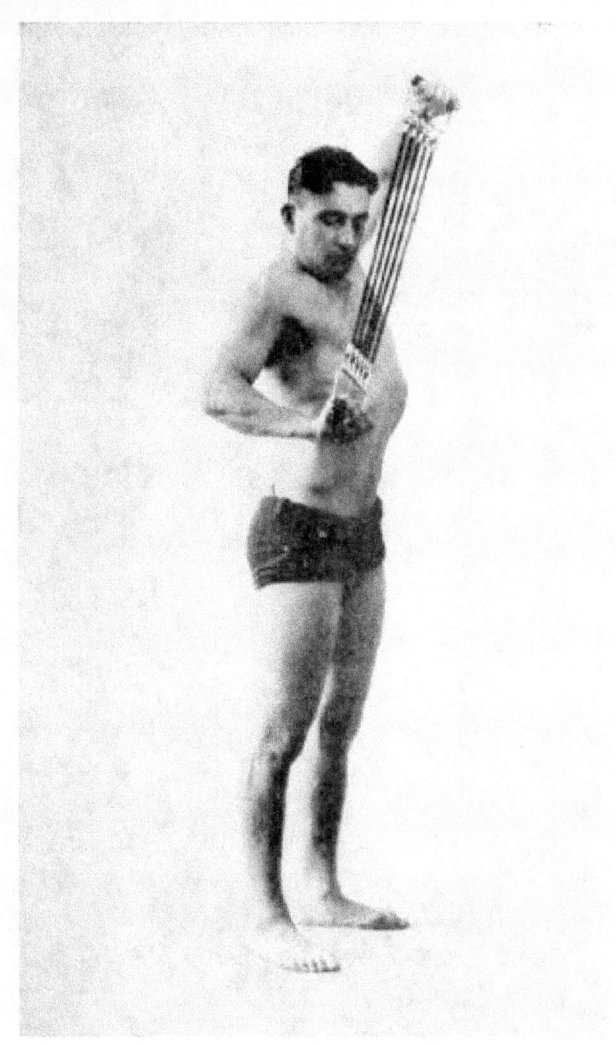

EXERCISE FOR THE ARMS

Hold exerciser in manner shown above. Left arm overhead and right arm bent. Then, push right arm downwards until arm is straight, still holding left arm overhead. An excellent exercise for the triceps. (See chapter on the arms.)

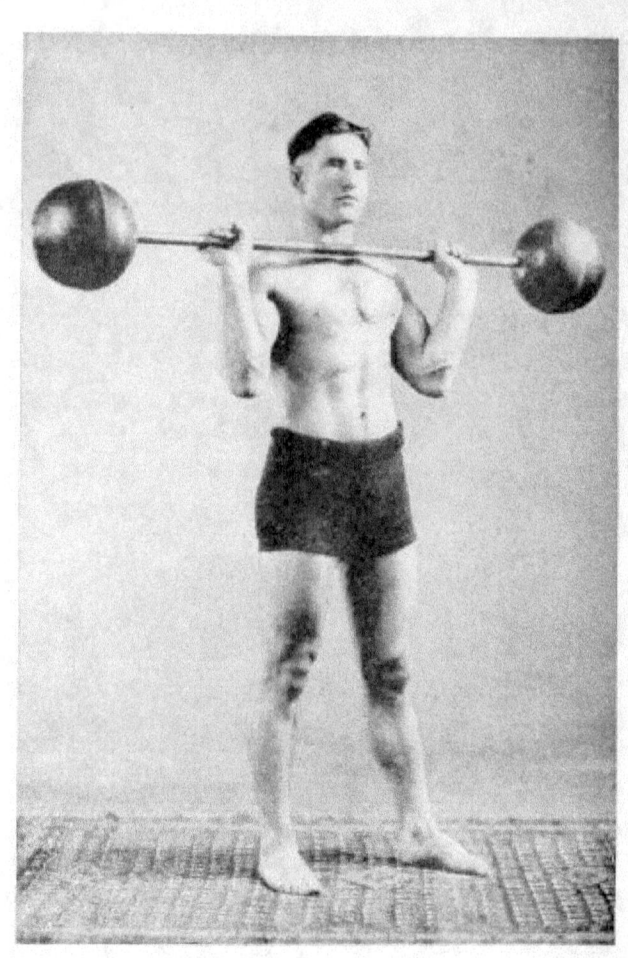

EXERCISE FOR THE ARMS

To exercise both arms at the same time, hold bar-bell at height of shoulders, as shown above.

* * *

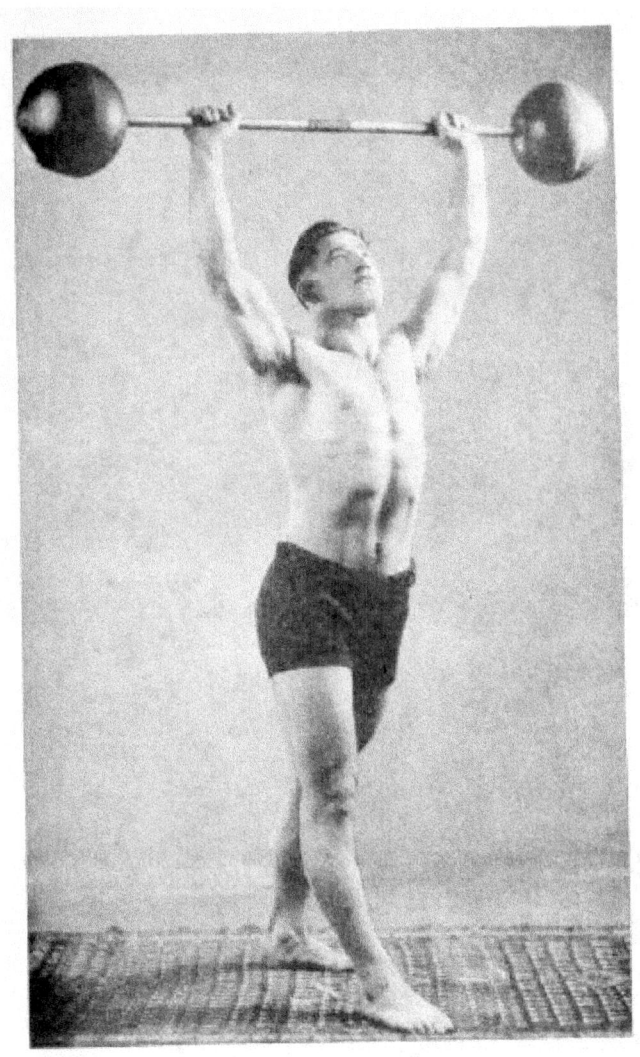

EXERCISE FOR THE ARMS

Then push bell upwards until both arms are stiff. (See chapter on the arms.)

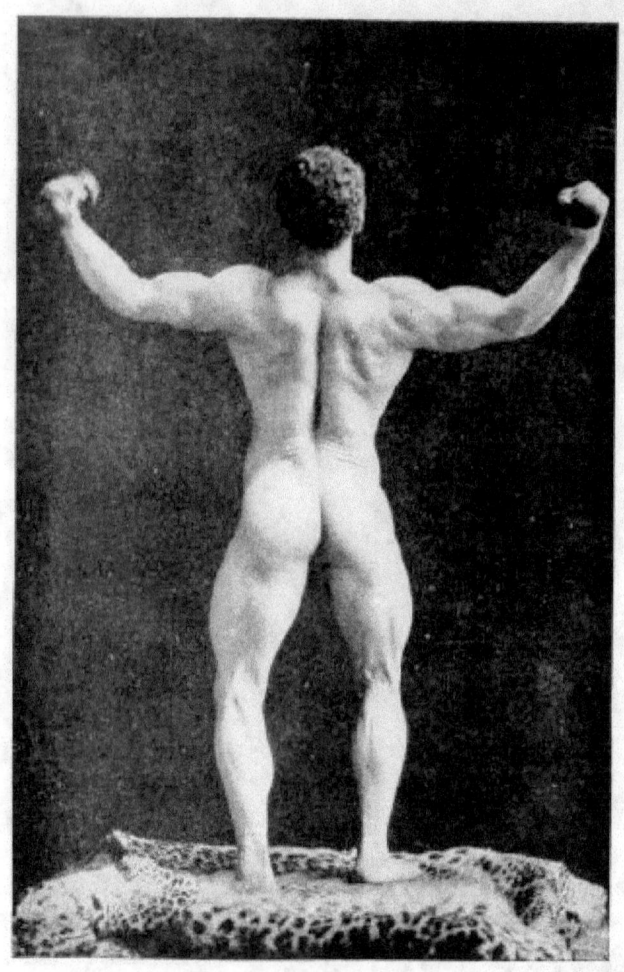

EXERCISE FOR THE ARMS

Eugen Sandow posed for the above photograph and is about to bring both bells to the shoulders at the same time. By using dumb-bells weighing from five to ten pounds in this movement, it will help greatly in adding finer tone to the biceps muscles. Be sure both arms are straightened between movements. (See chapter on the arms.)

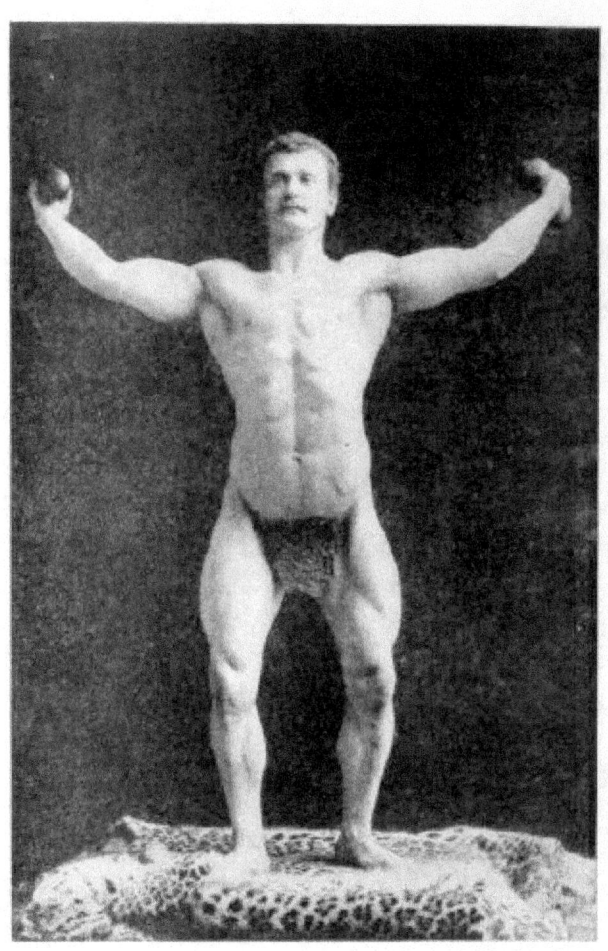

EXERCISE FOR THE ARMS

Hold both arms sideways, with firm grip on dumb-bells. (Mr. Sandow who posed for these photographs, was a firm believer in keeping the knees slightly bent throughout the entire exercise in order to give the thigh muscles some work at the same time.)

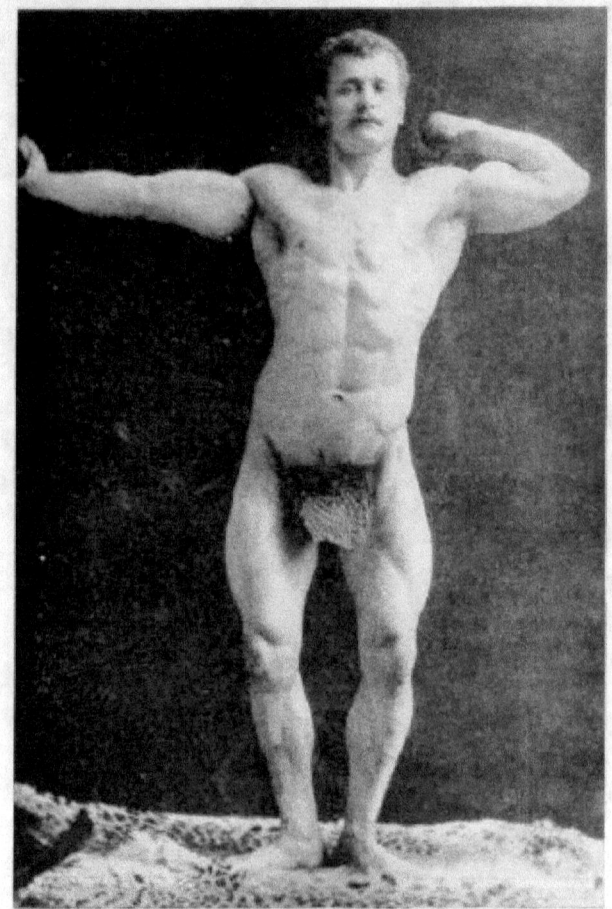

EXERCISE FOR THE ARMS

Then alternately bring one bell to shoulder. If light dumb-bell exercises are used in conjunction with heavier work, the arms will acquire better contour, especially in the biceps muscle. (See chapter on the arms.)

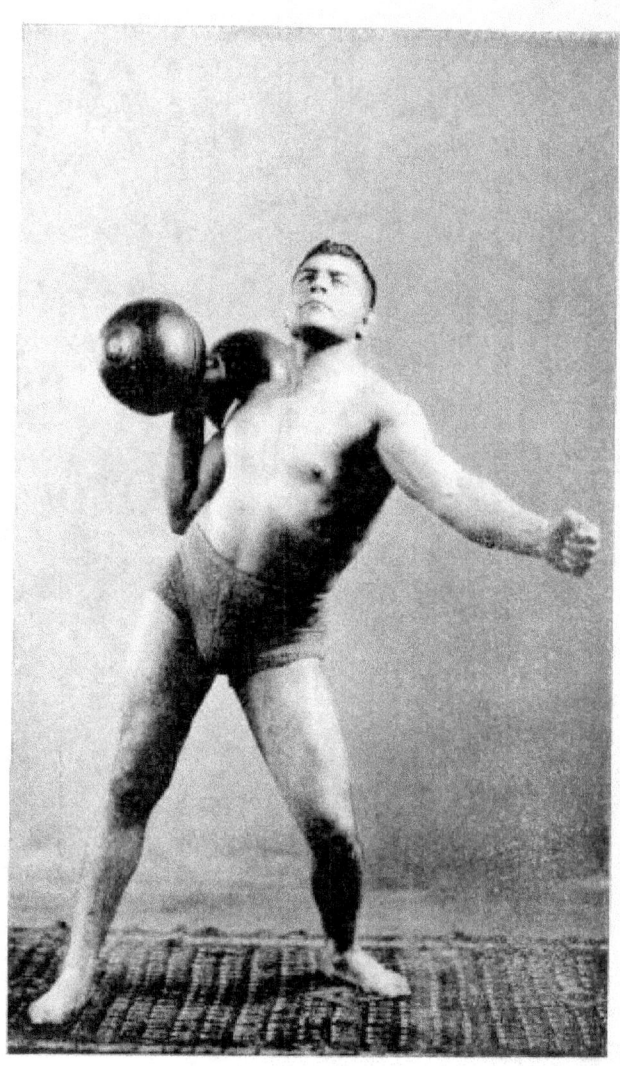

EXERCISE FOR THE ARMS

The start of the bent press. Hold bell at shoulder with right arm and place most of your weight on left leg. Twist forward with your left side and then start to bend sideways.

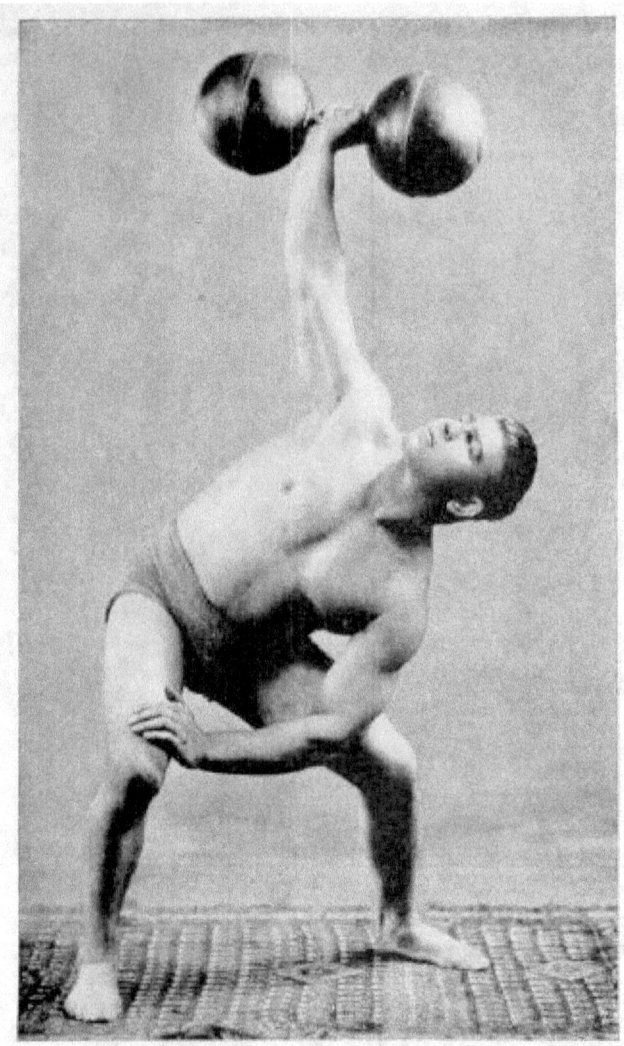

EXERCISE FOR THE ARMS

The action is not to push the bell upwards, but to move your body away from the weight. After bending sideways until arm is straight, the attempt should be made to stand erect with the bell. Assistance with the left hand or arm, as shown above, will help the lifter. The bent press is the only manner in which very heavy weights can be lifted overhead. (See chapter on the arms.)

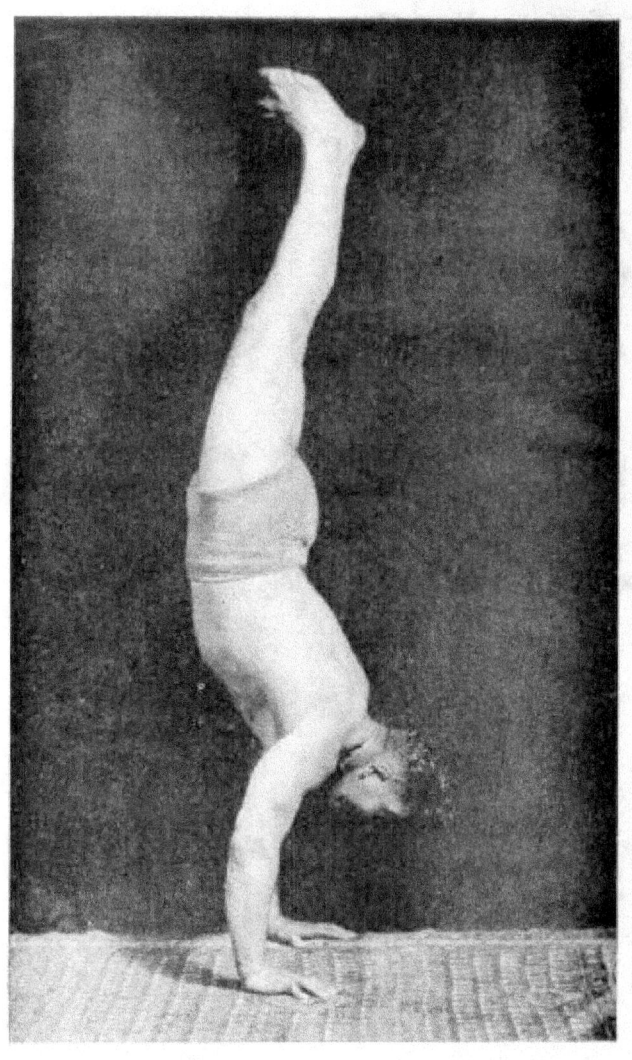

EXERCISE FOR THE ARMS

Hand balancing is an excellent pastime for one who desires strong arms. To further the arm development, dipping should be done while in the hand balance. Stand on hands as shown above.

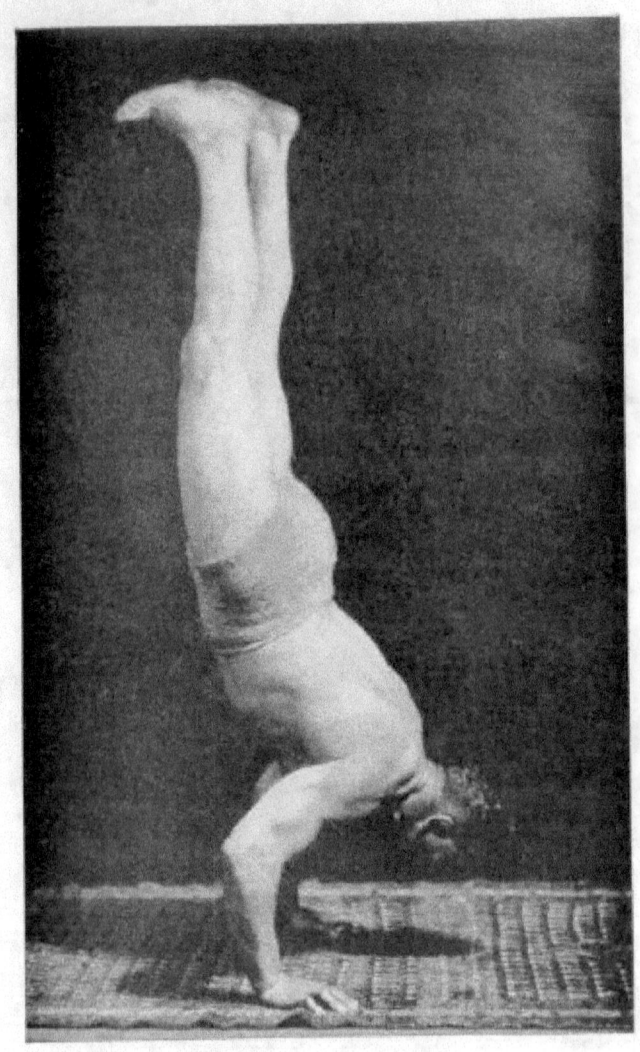

Exercise for the Arms

*Then lower chin to the floor and push up again until arms are straight.
An athlete who can perform a dozen dips in this manner has pretty
strong arms. (See chapter on the arms.)*

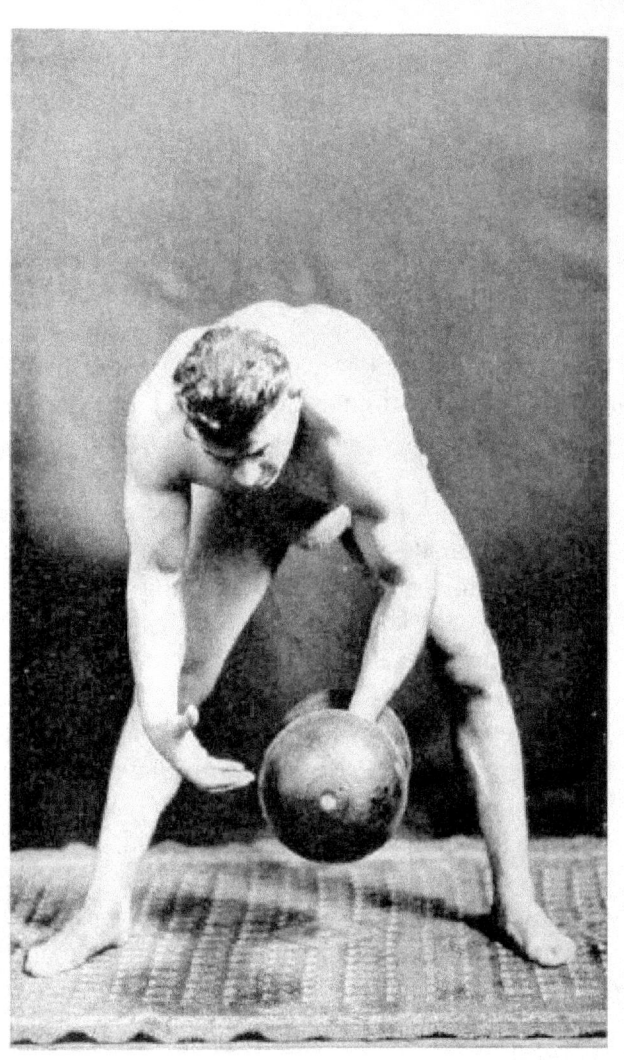

EXERCISE FOR THE ARMS

There are numerous exercises for the forearms, but one of the best consists of juggling a dumb-bell as shown above. Throw bell from one hand to the other until forearms ache. (See chapter on the arms.)

Chapter VIII
Training Your Abdomen to Make You Healthy

I WAS giving a series of lectures on physical culture some years ago in Chicago when a young doctor, who was some kind of a teacher in a medical college, took exception to a statement I made concerning the influence of exercise on health.

The doctor, who was pretty well married to the idea that the only way you could get relief from sickness was to take something out of a bottle, or else swallow a couple of pills, said:

"Mr. Liederman, do you mean to say that if a person takes exercise that he won't get sick; or if he is sick, that you can help him to get well by having him take exercises?"

I said: "I don't make any foolish claims to the effect that you can prevent all kinds of sickness by putting the body in perfect physical condition. Nor do I mean to say that all forms of sickness can be overcome by having a man take the right kind of exercises, for there are many kinds of sickness that are the result of direct infection.

"I do mean to say, however, that if a man will put himself into A1 physical condition by the proper kind of exercises and right living, that he stands a very small chance of ever developing any of the chronic ailments due to disorders of digestion and metabolism and the lack of proper elimination, that constitute nine-tenths of the doctor's business today.

"And I mean further to say, that even if he does contract acute diseases from infection, exposure, or other causes, that he'll get well about five times as fast if he is in fine physical shape as he would if he is all out of condition, from lack of proper physical exercise and failure to observe the essential rules of hygiene which I teach."

The doctor listened to what I had to say, and when I got through, he said: "Mr. Liederman, I take it all back. I see that what you have to say is founded on strict common sense. You win."

And this is now rapidly becoming the attitude of physicians all over the world. They are giving less and less medicine, and paying more and more attention to diet, hygiene, fresh air and exercise. And they're doing their patients infinitely more good than they ever did before, as a consequence.

The Abdominal Muscles and Their Importance

From the standpoint of health, there is no doubt that the abdominal muscles are the most important of all the muscles in the body—except, of course, the heart muscles. For the condition of the abdominal muscles either makes or mars the function of all the digestive organs, as well as the most important organs of elimination, the bowels.

Strong, well-developed waist muscles that hold the abdominal organs up in position and that prevent the sagging or prolapse that interferes so disastrously with their function, are absolutely essential to everyone who wants to remain in good health.

Therefore, I urge you to pay particular attention to the development of the muscles of the waist, so that you may enjoy the better health which development of the abdominal muscles brings about.

Now, to the average person the waist consists of two sizes, small and large. To the student of anatomy, however, there are as many variations in the waist as there are faces in the street. There are also long waists and short waists. The longer waisted individual usually has more endurance and more flexibility than a person who has a short waistline. In the trained athlete the waist usually presents its best appearance at about twenty-five years of age, for after that, there is a tendency to accumulate flesh, regardless of what physical training an individual may do.

This change may merely be a gain of an inch or two, but, nevertheless, after twenty-five years of age, the waist is never as small. Before the age of twenty, you very seldom see the muscles of the waist as thoroughly developed as they are after a man has reached his full growth, for, as a rule, the youthful waistline has a tendency to go in at the sides, where the external oblique abdominus muscle lies. Later on, when the boy commences training of the trunk region, the waist assumes a square appearance, owing to the pleasing development of the external oblique muscles.

The first muscle to show its appearance when the student performs a few weeks of abdominal work is the rectus abdominus. This muscle covers the front of the abdominal region, and when highly developed has a washboard appearance of eight fleshy digitations. If not developed to the maximum there are only six showing.

A Wonderful Specimen of Abdominal Development

One of the finest examples of abdominal development I have ever seen is that of Eugen Sandow. His muscles are of unusual quality and contour and he possesses remarkable control of them. The constant contraction of these abdominal muscles helps greatly to bring them out. The most simple contraction is performed by bending slightly forward and pressing downward on the thighs with the hands. The next step is the isolation of the rectus abdominus.

This is performed by emptying the lungs of air, pressing downward and outward on the upper thighs with the hands, and at the same time drawing in the abdominal wall, causing a cavity on each side of these muscles. I have seen some remarkable controls in this region. The single isolation, that is, having one side of the rectus abdominus muscle contracted and the other side drawn in with the abdominal cavity, is undoubtedly the most phenomenal of any muscular control that can be accomplished.

The quickest way to gain flesh around the abdominal region is to make yourself comfortable, and the larger the waistline becomes the more the skin is placed upon a stretch, until the weight of the superfluous flesh in front of the waist becomes saggy and lower. It is a simple matter to accumulate extra weight around the waist, but it is a very hard matter to rid oneself of it, as you may possibly have already found out. If a person will be careful of his diet, does not sit too much, and makes a point of standing erect at all times, he need have very little fear of becoming fleshy around the waist, especially if he performs daily set-ups and trunk movements.

After Thirty-five You May Have to Fight Fat

After thirty or thirty-five years of age, fleshy accumulations not only in the front of the waist, but in the sides and back, as well as the hips, will gradually form rolls of fat that are much harder to get rid of than is the superfluous flesh that gathers in front of the waist. A person whose habits are sedentary must pay special attention to the side of his back, the side of his waist and the front of his abdomen, if he expects to retain a small waistline the remainder of his days. He also must be careful of his diet, if he is inclined to put on flesh.

The nervous type individual who is high-strung need have little fear of ever acquiring a large waist, and should be thankful for that reason. If, however, he will devote care and attention to the rest of his body, combined with systematic training, he will find his progress much easier, and will waste less energy in his progress than the person who has constantly to fight the accumulation of flesh around the abdomen. My idea of the type of waist an athlete should possess is clearly shown in the portrait of

George Hackenschmidt on page 36. The waist shown in his pose is square, well-developed and yet slim, at the same time long, thus giving him remarkable endurance, flexibility and perfectly functioning organs.

It is very difficult to set a standard of measurements for the waistline, for a great deal depends upon the height and frame-work of the individual. A person who has a large frame-work, naturally will have a much wider waist than his small-boned competitor. This width of the waist will naturally increase the size by a couple of inches. The smaller the waist is, the larger the chest appears, and the broader the shoulders look. A person who devotes a lot of attention to abdominal work need never have any fear of constipation, indigestion or other similar ailments so common to the ordinary public.

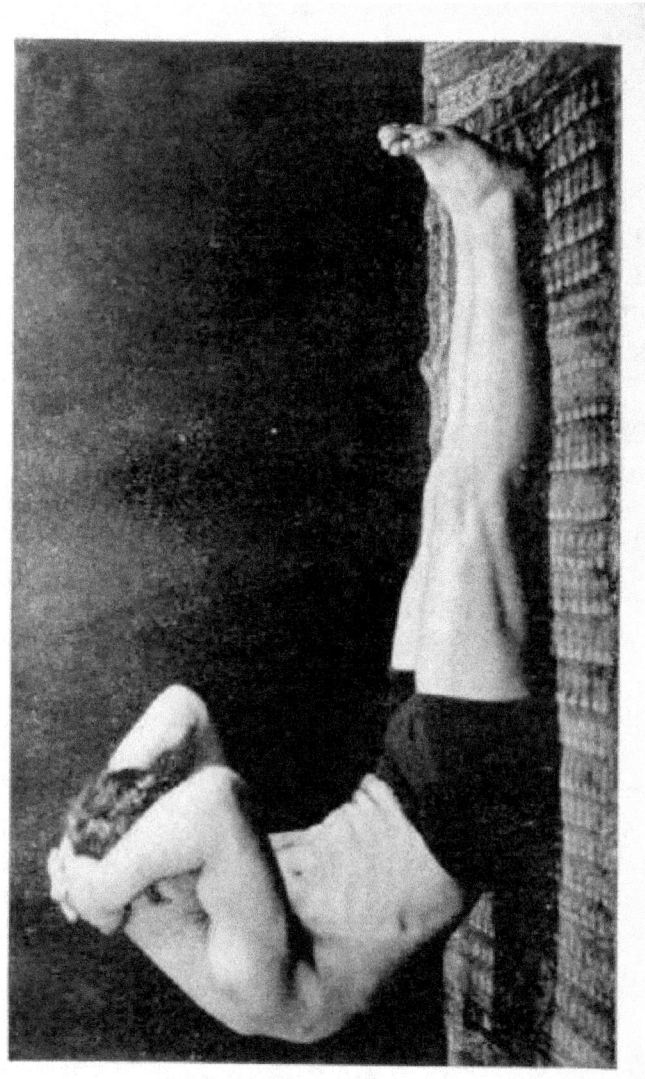

EXERCISE FOR THE ABDOMEN

Lie on your back, place hands behind head and then sit up until elbows touch knees. This is an excellent exercise for those who want to rid themselves of a large waist. (See chapter on abdomen.)

Exercises for the Waist

As I said before, the waistline to the obese individual is one of the most stubborn parts of the body to reduce, especially if considerable superfluous flesh is carried around the entire waist. The stout individual must work twice as hard as his slim neighbor if he expects to accomplish the same object, namely, a trim, square waist.

The same exercises that reduce the waist will build it up. This applies practically to every part of the body as well. A well-developed waistline is something everyone should strive for, as the prolonged efforts utilized to obtain waist symmetry will benefit and strengthen the digestive system, and make every organ function efficiently.

EXERCISE 1. One of the finest exercises for the waist is to lie on the floor and come to a sitting posture, while keeping the hands behind the head. The beginner may have to hook his feet under a dresser, couch or some other piece of furniture at first, to hold his feet down, but after a while he will be able to do this exercise without any difficulty.

The exercise should be continued until the muscles in the front part of the abdomen begin to feel uncomfortable. No special rules limiting the number of repetitions can be stipulated, because everyone is constituted differently, and too severe a strain upon the waist may cause hernia and other disagreeable strains; therefore, I do not advise the student to attempt to pick up weights while performing these exercises, or sitting up with these weights until he is well advanced in the work.

I suggest that the beginner do not attempt to perform more than ten repetitions for the first week or so, increasing gradually, until about twenty-five counts are reached. When he can do twenty-five repetitions after several months, he may pick up small objects of a few pounds or more, and perform this movement.

EXERCISE 2. Lie on your right side and raise both legs upward as high as possible, with the knees stiff. Lower the legs to the floor and repeat. This exercise is of special benefit for the sides of the waist, and should be performed until these waist muscles feel uncomfortable and start to ache. Do the same while lying on the opposite side.

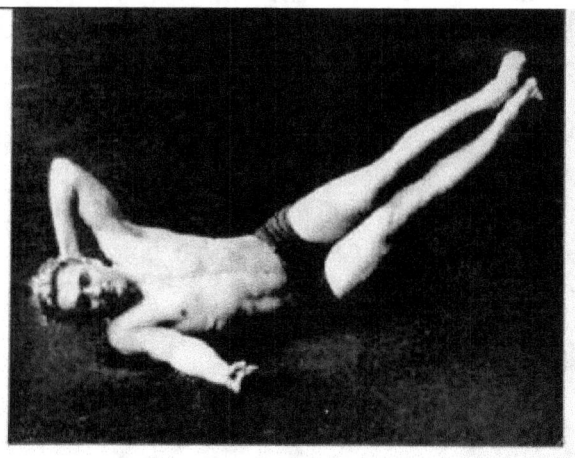

EXERCISE FOR THE ABDOMEN

Lie on floor on side and raise both legs sideways and upwards as shown above. (See chapter on abdomen.)

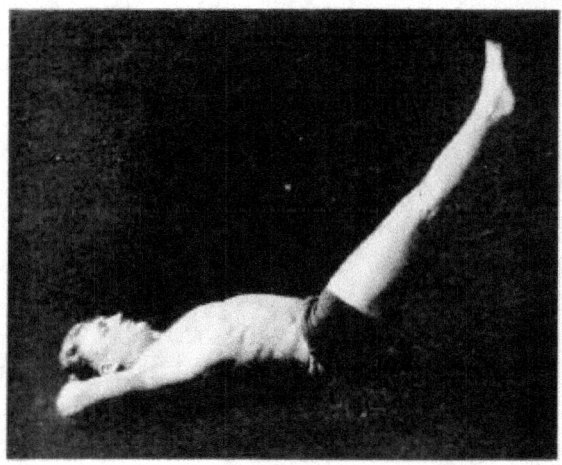

EXERCISE FOR THE ABDOMEN

Lie on back, raise both legs at height shown above. Then perform circles. First bring feet over head, then to side, then to floor, then to opposite side, until you have performed a complete circle. Unless legs are kept stiff throughout the entire exercise, you will get no direct benefit out of it.

162

EXERCISE 3. Lie on the back, and with knees stiff bring the legs as far as possible to the left, then upward as far as possible, then over to the right, until they almost touch the floor, then to the original starting position. This is called "leg circling," and is performed until the abdominal muscles feel uncomfortable. If you become tired, rest a minute and reverse the movement, until you become tired again.

EXERCISE 4. Raise the legs with knees stiff, and the arms with arms stiff, and touch the toe in mid-air while lying on your back. Lower to original position and repeat. Care should be taken each time when lowering that the body is completely outstretched on the floor, with the legs stiff and the hands extended overhead, otherwise, you will not get as much benefit out of this movement as you should. Continue until the abdominal muscles feel uncomfortable.

EXERCISE 5. While lying on your back, raise both legs upward and continue the movement until the toes touch the floor beyond your head. Return to original position and repeat until the abdominal region feels uncomfortable.

EXERCISE 6. While standing on the floor, raise arms overhead, and interlace the fingers, reaching upward as far as possible. While stretching in this position, bend as far as you can to the right, then as far as you can to the left. Continue until you feel tired at the sides of the waist or in the small of the back.

EXERCISE 7. Stand erect and reach upward as far as possible and clasp one hand with the other. Bend forward, keeping knees stiff, until your hands touch the floor. Raise upward again and bend backward as far as possible. These forward and backward movements you will find very suitable for warming-up exercises, before beginning heavier work.

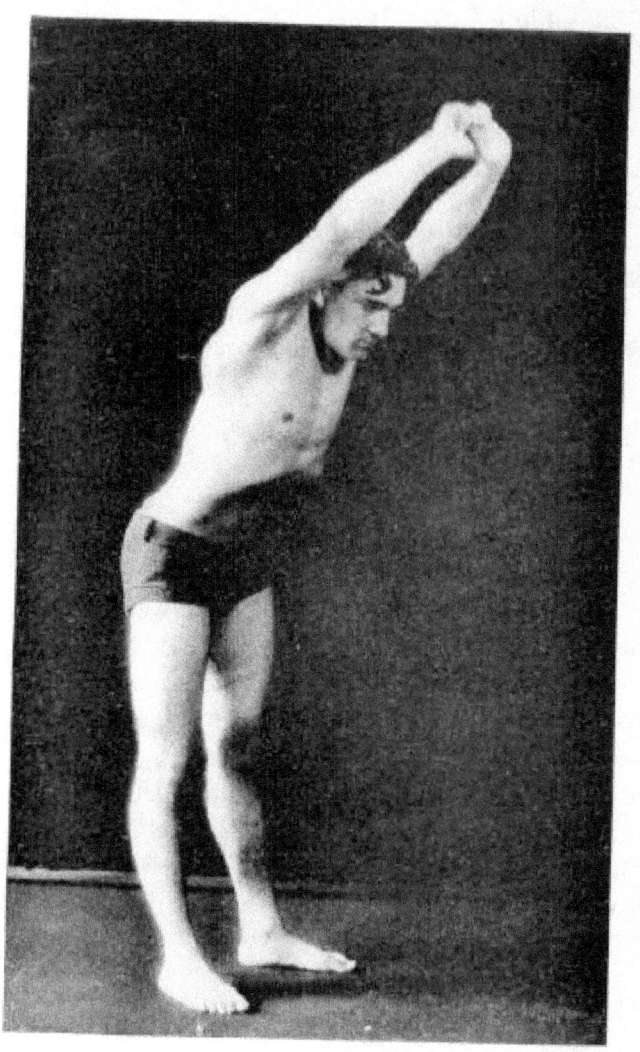

EXERCISE FOR THE ABDOMEN

Interlace hands overhead keeping arms stiff. Bend forward as shown above. (See chapter on abdomen.)

If the student will perform the exercises I have mentioned here, he will secure about all the abdominal work necessary for his day's drill. I do not believe in devoting too much time to the abdominal muscles, for if this is done, too much energy is used, thereby preventing attention to the muscle-building exercises, which are the subject of this book.

The abdominal muscles are exercised in conjunction with various other muscles in different exercises. However, direct application to abdominal movements is absolutely essential for health's sake, as well as in cases where superfluous flesh is carried around the waist, or where greater abdominal development is desired.

The student should do at least one or two abdominal exercises every day, such as sitting up, touching the toes, or sitting up with hands behind head in order to prevent any chance of superfluous flesh gathering around his waistline, and also to stimulate his internal organs.

The lifting of a bar-bell from the floor to the height of the waist and lowering again, which I mention in the development of the latissimus dorsi muscle, is of special benefit as well for the muscles of the lower back, where fat generally accumulates in sedentary individuals.

There is one thing I would like to emphasize before leaving this subject. The abdominal muscle exercises, above all others, are the one form of exercise you should never give up. For the older you get the more need you'll have for doing everything in your power to keep the abdominal organs functioning properly. And these are the exercises that will do the trick.

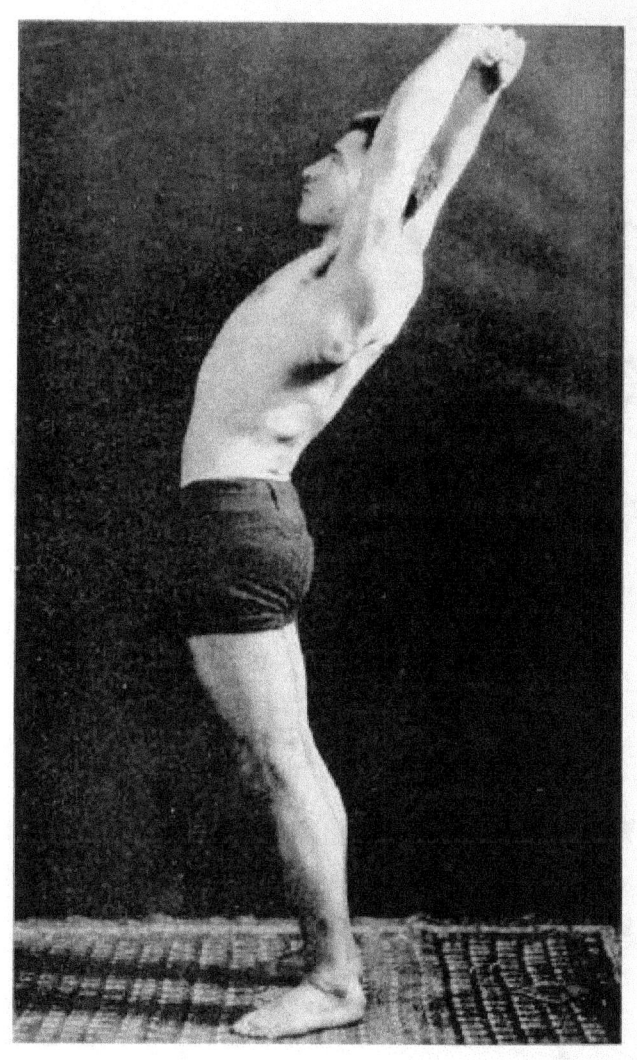

EXERCISE FOR THE ABDOMEN

Interlace hands overhead keeping arms stiff. Bend backwards as shown above. (See chapter on abdomen.)

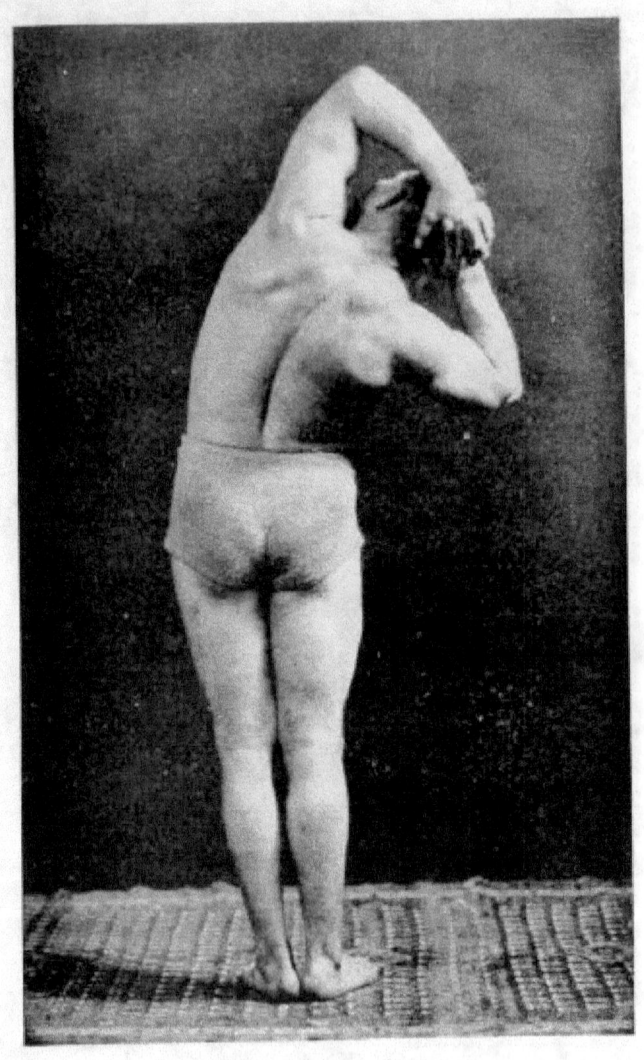

EXERCISE FOR THE ABDOMEN
Clasp hands behind head and bend from side to side as far as possible.
(See chapter on the abdomen.)

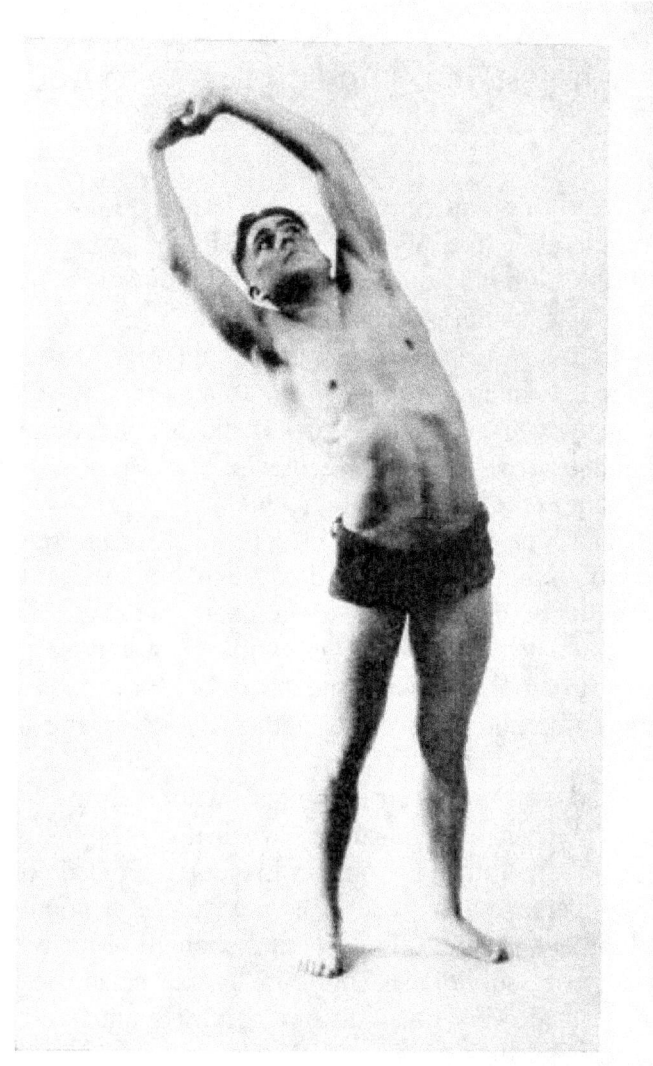

Chapter IX
Symmetrical Hips and How to Acquire Them

VERY little attention is generally paid to the hips by the average athlete in his course of training, owing to the fact that the formation of the male hips are of little consequence as far as personal pride is concerned.

If a boy or a young man should seem to show any particular interest in his hips, as an ordinary thing "the gang" would be inclined to kid the life out of him. This should not be so, because the hips are a very important element in the make-up of an athlete.

The hips vary greatly in appearance, and considerable attention should be devoted to them, because strong hips, with plenty of endurance, are a great asset to an individual. A person with wide hips naturally has a wide waist and a very strong frame-work and, therefore, is capable of great supporting and feats of strength in which strong hips play an important part.

The narrow-hipped individual, with a narrow waist, can never expect to be as strong, when it comes to displaying feats of strength and lifting, as his larger- framed competitor.

A person with wide hips usually has a good leg development, owing to the size and strength of his bones, and it is these individuals who, with proper scientific training, turn out to be not only the finest built athletes, but remarkably strong men as well.

Well-developed hips are essential, first, for endurance, as in running, walking, carrying heavy objects, climbing, etc., for it is in this part of the body that the first signs of fatigue are manifested in performing any of these exercises. The gluteus maximus, the largest muscle of the hip, when properly developed, gives a pleasing curve to the lower back, which is much more desirable than to see flabby tissue covering this part.

A well-trained athlete's hips usually are slightly hollow at the sides, and when contracted the gluteus maximus muscle is clearly shown. Most of the men who are "understanders," or "bottom men," in hand-balancing acts, have thoroughly developed hips. This comes naturally to them from the work they do, causing a great strain to be placed upon the hips in supporting their partner when doing hand-to-hand work.

The Powerful Hips of Arab Tumblers

Undoubtedly you have seen various troupes of tumbling Arabs or Japs. Possibly you have noticed that one of them, during their act, is able to support the entire troupe, who climb and pile upon him and around him. I have seen one act in particular of this nature, where a single man supported the weight of nine other men, and still was able to take a few walking steps with this enormous weight. If this man did not have exceptionally strong hips, and if his hips were not wide enough to give him exceptionally good support, this tremendous weight would cause him to collapse.

A wide-hipped man, being a heavier-boned man, as a rule, naturally is inclined to be of a heavy type, and will weigh more when in his highly developed state than an individual whose muscles are equally as well developed, but whose hips are narrow.

Exercises for the Hips

Undoubtedly the finest exercise to strengthen the hips is to walk while carrying heavy objects, especially while climbing stairs.

This is a very severe exercise and should not be undertaken until after you have developed a considerable amount of strength in the muscles of the hips and thighs.

I would suggest that you first practice stair-climbing, without carrying any weights. Let the arms hang loosely at the side, and do not try to pull yourself upstairs by holding on to the railing, or putting your hands against the wall.

After you have practiced this for a few weeks, and your strength and wind power are sufficiently developed, you might start by carrying weights, commencing with a light weight of 10 or 15 pounds, and gradually working up to it, until you can carry 50 pounds up three or four flights of stairs without any difficulty.

A great many movements can be performed for the hips, although the ones that have special merit are lateral work, such as lying on the floor on your side and raising first one leg, and then both legs, while keeping them stiff; also while lying on your stomach endeavoring to raise both legs upward, keeping the legs stiff.

Leg Circling

While lying on your back, by performing double leg circling, you give the hips quite a play. These circles should be made as wide as possible; that is, starting from a reclining position on your back and keeping the legs stiff, bring both feet as far as you can to the left and then upward and backward over your head, and then as far as you can to the right, until they almost touch the floor. Then return to original position. All these movements should be reversed in order to work the muscles in the opposite direction. I mentioned all this in the chapter on the abdomen, but repeat it again here, for this circling exercise applies to the hips as well.

Another excellent exercise for developing the hips is to stand on both feet, then raise the right leg with the knee stiff to a horizontal position, where it will be at right angles out in front of the body. Swing your arms up level with your shoulders, in order to keep your balance. Then lower the leg slowly and bring it up again, as often as you can, until the hips are tired. You should not do this too quickly or with any evidence of a jerk, for it is the contraction and lift of the muscles, and not the momentum of the swing, that secures the results you are aiming at in this particular exercise.

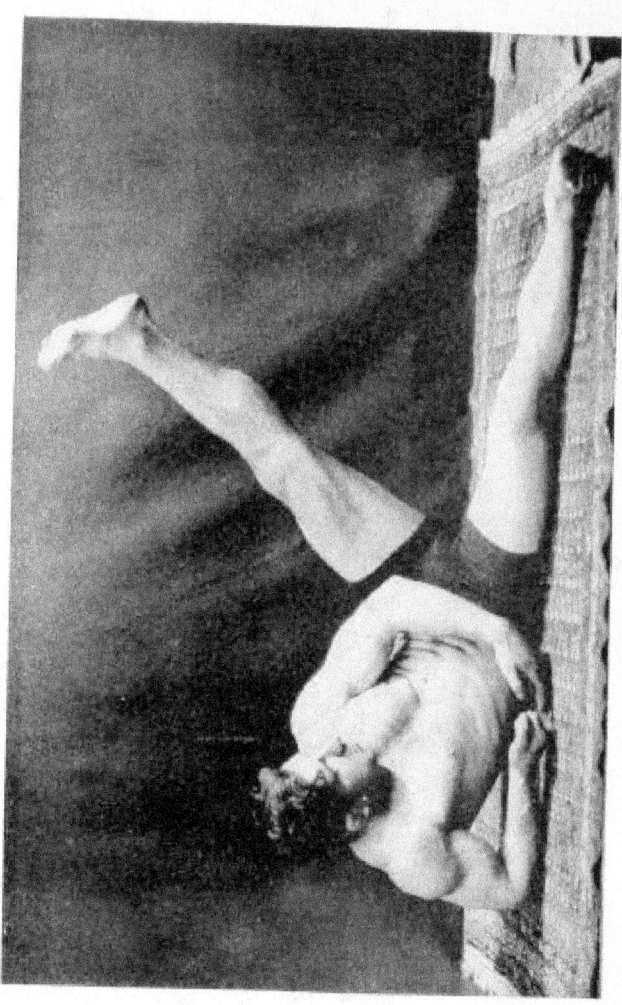

EXERCISE FOR THE HIPS

Lie on floor on side and raise legs sideways and upwards as shown above. (See chapter on the hips.)

Rest for a minute or two, and then repeat the exercise, using the left leg this time, until tired.

Then rest a while, and do this same exercise, extending the legs out to the side this time, instead of straight ahead. This is more difficult than the forward lift, and you will not be able to do it so often before becoming fatigued. However, it is very important, because it brings into play different hip muscles than are stressed in the preceding exercise. Use both legs alternately, as before.

After a short rest, stand as before, and raise the legs straight backward, bringing each leg up as high as possible and holding the position a second or two, so as to get the greatest amount of good from it.

Good for the Fat and the Lean

These exercises are just as good for taking off excess fat as they are for building up solid muscle—in fact, you've got to get rid of your fat before you really can put solid muscle on.

So, if you are too fat, don't be surprised to see the size of your hips reduced within a month or so, possibly by several inches. This, however, is only preliminary to building up firm, well-developed muscle, that will be of great value to you in all feats of strength, and that will serve to give your entire body much better developed and more symmetrical lines.

If you are thin and underweight, on the other hand, you will find that, after a few weeks of these exercises, you'll be conscious of a very definite increase in development.

I emphasize this matter very strongly because a great deal depends upon your hip development, if you are to bring out the general contour of your figure, and have the symmetrical lines of a perfect athlete.

Chapter X
The Well-developed Thigh

THE thighs, when properly developed, are undoubtedly the most beautiful sets of muscles of which the human body can boast. A well-rounded, highly developed pair of thighs will put a professional finished touch on any athlete.

Well-shaped thighs are most notable on all professional strong men, especially tumblers and weight lifters, for such physical work places direct application on the quadriceps extensor muscles, which constitute the group of muscles covering the entire front and sides of the thighs. Again I am forced to admit that Eugen Sandow had perhaps the finest contour of this group of muscles that I have ever seen.

However, the most remarkable pair of thighs, so far as size is concerned, were owned by William Gerardi, whose thighs measure, I believe, over 31 inches. (See page 26.)

Sprinters and Jumpers Usually Have Great Thigh Development

Sprinters have exceptionally developed thighs, produced by the heavy exertion of their speedy work. However, endurance runners, as a rule, are lacking greatly in leg development, as the muscles are overworked. Consequently the tissues are destroyed faster than they can be replenished. It is a known and proven fact that prolonged repetition of movement, when carried to the point of absolute fatigue and even beyond that, to exhaustion, causes the muscles to wear away. Therefore, many well-developed athletes are now dead from the effects of prolonged fatiguing exercises.

The student need have no fear, however, or be frightened by the above statement, for the strength of the muscles will be ever on the increase, as long as he discontinues the movement when the aching point is reached. At this point you should thoroughly relax and allow the blood to flow freely while in this relaxed state. After a short period of rest, resume your work until the muscles ache again, thus tiring them for the second time during the exercise period. In this way you will make most rapid progress.

The Kind of Exercise Makes a Great Difference

The kind of exercise that the thighs are called upon to perform has a great deal to do with the size and shape of the muscles to be developed. I have found from experience that slow, heavy work is best to develop the quadriceps extensor muscles. The position of the feet must also be taken into consideration. When the feet are placed flat on the floor with the toes pointed outward, the legs somewhat spread apart, say about 18 inches or more, and deep knee-bending is performed (whether this be done with a heavy weight on the shoulders or against some powerful resistance), the sartorious muscle is brought into play. This muscle, when developed, fills in the space usually seen in poorly developed legs under the crotch, and gives not only strength, but a pleasing curve to the inside of the thighs.

The sartorious muscle is also known as the "tailor's muscle." This term was given it owing to the practice of old-time tailors who sat on the floor, and raised themselves with legs crossed and without the help of the hands, relying only on the strength of this muscle.

The vastus internus and the vastus externus, as well as the rectus femoris are the remaining three muscles that give the curve from the knee to the hip, on the inside and on the outside of the thigh. These muscles can be developed to some extent by the common deep knee-bending exercise, but if the student desires exceptional development and extraordinary curves, he must perform this deep knee-bending exercise against a powerful resistance, or else with some heavy weight on his shoulders.

The feet should be parallel with each other when performing this exercise, for the greatest strain is placed directly upon the thighs if the heels are kept flat on the floor. If the heels are raised from the floor, the lower legs or calf muscles are required to share some of the burden.

The Shape of the Legs Largely Inherited

Heredity has a lot to do with the size of the legs. Some people are naturally fortunate in having fairly well-developed legs, without any exercise whatever, while others possess legs that are exceedingly thin and ungainly. A person who inherits a good-sized leg has everything in his favor in attempting to convert the flesh into good, solid muscle—and well-formed muscle at that.

However, a person whose legs are thin need not be discouraged, for scientifically applied exercise will give anyone the curves and the strength that he desires. Of course, the small-boned man again must not expect to obtain the strength and the bulk of his heavier-boned competitor. The fact has been proven in hundreds and hundreds of cases of small-boned athletes, whose thighs were exceptionally developed, that the small-boned man has just as much of an incentive to work for, and even more than a heavy-framed individual.

The thighs play an important part in feats of strength, and work in unison with the muscles of the hips, especially in performing lifts and in carrying and working with heavy objects. The common exercise of deep knee-bending is a very good one to begin with for improvement of the thighs. However, I would not advise its continuance except as a warming-up exercise, after a period of about three months, for then the thighs are in a state to receive heavier work.

The student should then endeavor to perform deep knee-bending on one leg, or run upstairs two or three steps at a time, thereby giving the thighs additional work. After a month or two of this, you should adopt more vigorous methods, if you expect further improvement in the thigh muscles.

Don't Neglect the Biceps of Your Leg

One of the most sadly neglected muscles in the body is the biceps femoris, below the buttocks in the back of the thigh. This muscle contracts the leg and is an exceedingly stubborn one to develop. Sprinters as a rule are well developed in this part. But in order to develop this muscle to its limit, one has to resort to special exercises.

The lifting of heavy objects from the floor while bending over and keeping the knees stiff, and then bringing the object to the waist, while straightening up to an erect position, will place pressure upon this biceps femoris muscle. Unless this muscle is properly developed the thighs lack the finishing touches of harmonious development.

Next time you attend the theatre, pay particular attention to the acrobats, the strong men or the dancers, and if you are fortunate enough to see these men's legs either with or without tights on, you will have an excellent opportunity of noting what a vast improvement a beautiful curve behind the thigh makes in the appearance of the legs.

Classical dancing will also develop this muscle. The juggling of a weight placed on your foot and held in an upright position while lying on your back, will also develop the leg biceps. The common limbering-up exercise practiced by toe dancers, which consists in grasping the heel and raising the leg forward and upward, until the knee is stiff, will also put a strain upon this muscle, and help its development.

In practicing exercises for the thigh you must be exceedingly careful in the beginning and not put too much strain upon the legs or hips, or work with too much enthusiasm. For harmful results, such as a rupture, might come from such thoughtlessness. Progress gradually; do not be impatient and expect to see results all at once. You must never try to lift heavy objects until your legs are somewhat developed, and capable of the extra strain. Then when you do, be sure that you stand pigeon-toed; that is, with the toes inclined to turn toward each other. Never stand with the toes pointed outward when lifting heavy objects. For when the toes are pointed outward, the strain is placed mostly on the sartorious and adductor muscles, and too great a strain on these muscles may prove serious. When the toes are pointed inward, the strain is placed on the vastus internus and vastus externus muscles of this quadriceps extensor group.

Exercises for the Thighs

As I said before, the ordinary deep knee-bending exercise is a good one for beginners to use as a limbering-up movement, but it is much too light an exercise to yield any marked results in development. It won't be long before you will be able to squat down and up hundreds of times. Instead of adding strong muscular tissues on your thighs, you will tear the tissues down quicker than they can be replenished, by overwork.

Although the thighs should really be worked similarly to the arms and shoulders; that is, tiring the extensor muscles within ten repetitions, nevertheless, caution should be used in performing leg work, owing to the fact that overstraining may result in hernia. I, therefore, suggest that the student perform at least twenty or twenty-five repetitions, in order to tire the muscles thoroughly. In order to get the quadriceps extensor muscles aching in twenty-five counts, artificial resistance must be resorted to.

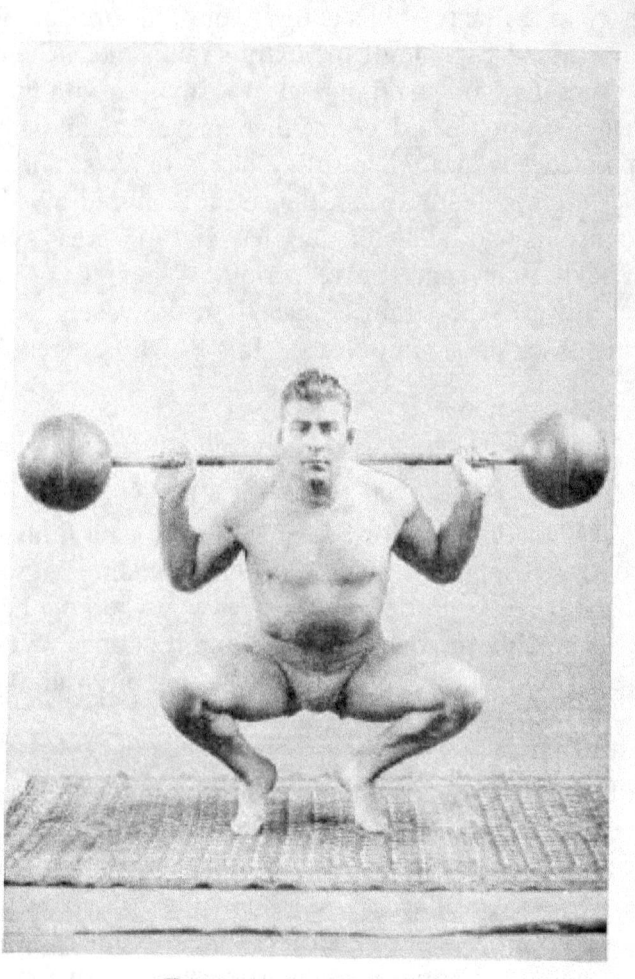

EXERCISE FOR THE THIGHS

Place bar-bell on shoulders and perform the deep knee-bending exercise as shown above. Squat as far downwards as possible, then come to a standing position. This exercise can be varied by performing the movement on the toes as the model has done, or by keeping the feet flat on the floor—thus working the thigh muscles in a slightly different manner. (See chapter on the thighs.)

The best means of securing additional resistance for these exercises is to place a bar-bell upon the shoulders. Perform the deep knee-bending exercises with this weight adjusted to suit the strength of your legs. If you are good for twenty-five repetitions, and your muscles do not ache as much as they did in the beginning, you should increase the weight. If you have no weight I suggest you perform the deep knee-bending exercise on one leg at a time. In this manner, you will be able to tire your muscles more readily.

To make the movement still more difficult without the use of a weight, you can step up on the edge of a table until you are standing in an erect position. Then lower yourself again, until one leg touches the floor. This gives the muscles a little more work than if you performed a one-leg deep knee-bend on the floor.

There is still another method of developing the thighs, if the student has no bar-bell. That is, to have someone sit on your shoulders, straddling your neck, and perform your deep knee-bending exercise that way. Progress can be made by having heavier and heavier individuals help you out.

When performing deep knee-bending with bar-bell or with someone sitting on your shoulders, keep the feet flat on the floor. Do not raise the heels off the floor when reaching the squatting position. This will enable you to squat further down and almost sit on the floor, thereby giving complete contractions and extensions to your muscles. Keep your toes pointed front and your feet about 12 inches apart.

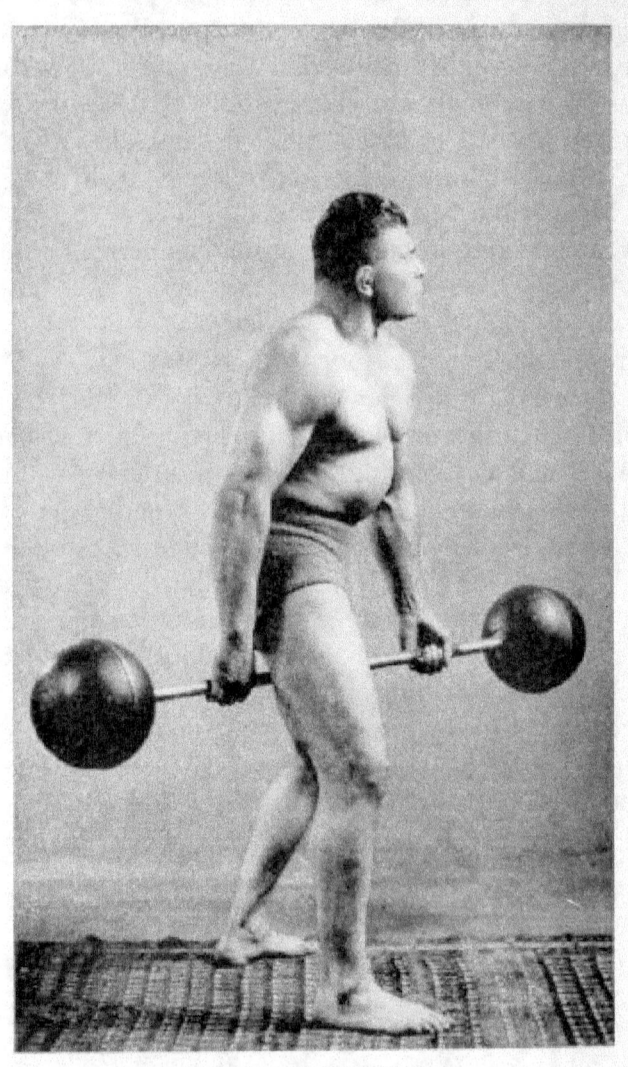

EXERCISE FOR THE THIGHS

Straddle bar-bell as shown above. Then perform a half squat. This movement plays upon the inside of the thighs. (See chapter on the thighs.)

A Great Exercise with the Bar-bell

Another exercise that will greatly build up the belly of the extensor muscles and, at the same time, give strong play to the sartorious muscle, is as follows:

Stand with feet about 20 inches apart or more, depending upon the length of your legs. Then, with a weight on your shoulders, and toes pointed outward, with feet flat on the floor, perform a half-squat, that is, bend the knees about half way. This can also be done with a bar-bell held with both hands between your crotch. In performing this movement, be sure to keep the body erect and tire the muscles within twenty-five repetitions. Care should be taken by the beginner in this exercise not to use too heavy a weight or resistance. For when the toes are pointed outward, there is more danger of a strain or hernia than when the toes are pointing straight forward, or even inward. However, you need not fear a strain if you go about it systematically and do not let your ambitions and enthusiasm get the better of you.

Almost every athlete who has well-developed legs also has an excellent lung capacity, for you cannot develop the legs without developing the lungs at the same time. You will find this out for yourself as you progress with the work. It will be a good thing to do a little breathing exercise after you have finished your leg work, for then you will be out of breath, and when you are out of breath, deep breathing will do you a world of good.

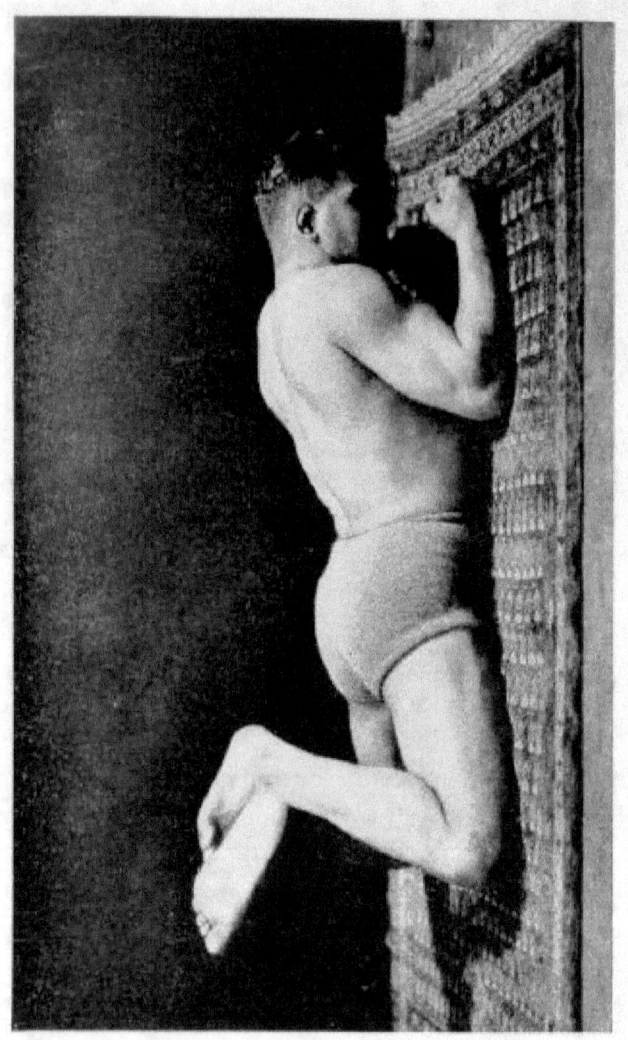

EXERCISE FOR THE THIGHS

The biceps of the leg, being a sadly neglected muscle, and little used as well, needs direct application in order to bring out its curve. An excellent exercise consists of lying face down on the floor and crossing feet as shown above. Next endeavor to straighten the legs by pushing against one foot with the other, resisting meanwhile with the antagonistic muscles. (See chapter on the thigh.)

Exercising the Leg Biceps

The muscle behind the thighs, known as the biceps of the legs, as I told you previously, is a sadly neglected muscle and is very seldom prominent, even on many professional athletes. There are dozens of movements that you can perform to work this muscle, but here are two of the best. Bend over with the knees stiff and pick up a heavy weight from the floor, bring it to an erect position in front of you, and lower again. Repeat this until the muscles at the back of the legs are distinctly tired. Lie on your stomach, bending your knees until your heels almost touch your hips, and push one leg with the other until your legs are straight, forcing yourself to work against as much resistance as your legs will permit.

Also, in picking up a bar-bell from the floor, exercise should be made progressive as you become stronger in the leg biceps, by standing on books or low stools and picking the weights up from the floor, with the knees stiff. If you bend your knees at all in this exercise, you lose the most important part of it.

By keeping the knees stiff at all times, you will feel the strain directly upon the biceps of the legs. The simple exercise of bending over and touching the floor with the palms of your hands, without bending your knees, also affects this muscle, but you will not make much progress by continuing this light movement. You should progress in this exercise until you are able to stand on a strong chair that will not tip over, and with the bar-bell held in front of you, bend over with knees stiff until the weight hangs down below your feet as far as possible, and then straighten up again as far as possible. By adjusting the resistance you work against, you should very easily tire your leg biceps muscle within twenty-five repetitions, or even less.

In the exercise where you lie on your stomach and resist with your legs, you must concentrate strongly on this movement. Otherwise, the amount of resistance you work against will become lighter and lighter, in which case you will not progress very rapidly.

Lying on your back and juggling a bar-bell placed on your feet when your feet are extended upward, will also benefit this muscle. But I do not advise this exercise except to advanced students who have become used to handling a bar-bell. For the beginner is liable to allow the bell to slip off his feet and fall on him, thereby resulting in an injury.

Short sprints will also benefit the thigh muscles, for they put direct strain on these muscles and give them definite work to do. However, as I said when speaking of the hips—and the same thing applies to the thighs— if you want to be a developed athlete, with a well-rounded physique, perfect in all its proportions, don't neglect your hips and thighs. For lack of care in exercising these muscles will be apparent, at first glance, to any trainer or teacher of physical culture, and will inevitably detract from the harmonious appearance your body would otherwise have.

Chapter XI
The Calf and Its Sturdy Curve

A SHORT time ago I was at a gathering at which there were several famous stage beauties, who were known for their devotion to physical culture. The discussion naturally turned toward physical culture and its influence on health and beauty, which was admitted by everybody.

Finally, one of the ladies, known to every theatregoer for her wonderful ability as a dancer, turned to me and said:

"Mr. Liederman, there's one thing that has always impressed me on the bathing beaches. There isn't one man in a thousand who hasn't ugly legs. Either they are too fat, or they are too stringy and skinny.

"You may see hundreds of girls with beautifully formed legs, calves and ankles, but you very seldom see a man who would pass muster, especially from his knees down. Why is this?"

I replied that very few men pay any attention to symmetrical development, or muscle building. They try to build up a big chest, or shoulders or arms. But they hardly ever give a thought to their lower extremities. These leg muscles, do not show so much for the work put in on their development. Again, the means used to bring about this development are practically unknown, except to a few physical culture specialists—who have paid particular attention to building up these ordinarily stringy muscles into well-rounded proportions.

The Calf of the Leg Hard to Develop

As a matter of fact, the calf of the leg is, without doubt, one of the hardest parts of the body to develop, owing to the fact that the muscle is continually placed in a contracted state by walking, and the further fact that it responds very slowly to exercise. The size and shape of the calf, the same as with the thigh, depends greatly upon heredity. Some people fortunately possess well-shaped legs below the knee, while others less fortunate have great difficulty in developing the muscles of the calf even to fair proportions.

A person with an exceptionally developed pair of calves, regardless of what some people may claim, must, in the first place, have had a certain amount of fleshy tissue to begin with. Then, with considerable muscle- building work, he will be able to develop the gastrocnemius muscle behind the calf to exceptional proportions.

Again, the length of the bone must be taken into consideration. The tall individual with long bones cannot develop a calf in proportion to a chap whose legs are short. Therefore, you usually find phenomenal calf development among people of somewhat short stature. In order to give his calves the proper amount of attention the lanky individual has to do double the amount of work that the fellow who begins with a little beef in this part of his anatomy has to do.

The common exercise of rising up and down on the toes will start the student off with calf development. However, he cannot expect to develop to any marked degree by this light exercise. Therefore, after a few weeks, he should resort to rising up and down on the toes on one leg at a time. He will then have to progress again after a short period by working the calves against a stronger resistance, and keep on progressing.

The calves should be tired at least two or three times during each exercise period. The student need have little fear of overstraining the muscles of the calf, because they are capable of supporting great strain.

The calves are one of the first places varicose veins put in their appearance. These are caused by continual standing on the feet, thereby keeping the muscles in an over-tensed state, and consequently causing the walls of the veins and arteries to become weakened.

To the average student the gastrocnemius muscle, or the muscle behind the calf, constitutes the main object of lower leg development. In reality, however, a muscle of vital importance is the muscle of the shin, for this muscle, when properly developed, gives the calf 50 per cent, more attention value, and changes the appearance of the outside and front of the calf.

Size of the Ankle a Great Factor

The size of the ankle has a great deal to do with the shape of the calf. A person who has small ankles will undoubtedly have better shaped legs than a person whose ankles are thick and heavy. It is a peculiar thing, and one that very few people seem to know anything about, but persons with thick ankles are usually subject to weak ankles. The slim-ankled individual hardly ever develops sprains or strains in this part.

Much of what I have said regarding the development of the muscles of the thighs and the hips applies with almost equal force to the calves. Running, jumping, and climbing are especially valuable. I also recommend rope skipping, especially when you spring from the toes with each skip, as this puts direct strain on the muscle of the calf.

It goes without saying that this exercise is also splendid for lung development and for increasing wind and endurance. I also recommend dancing as a good exercise for developing the calves, especially if you'll "stay up on your toes" as much as you can, and not slouch into the lazy habit of spending most of your time on the soles of your feet.

I do not believe it is possible to over-emphasize the importance of development of the muscles of the calves in bringing about a more springy and elastic stride when walking, and even a moderate amount of weakness or lack of development in the calf muscles will diminish the grace and freedom of your walk. This springiness is one of the first things you lose when the arches of your feet break down. And the lack of the power and development that brings about this springiness, is in turn one of the chief evidences of that relaxation of the muscles that finally results in flat feet.

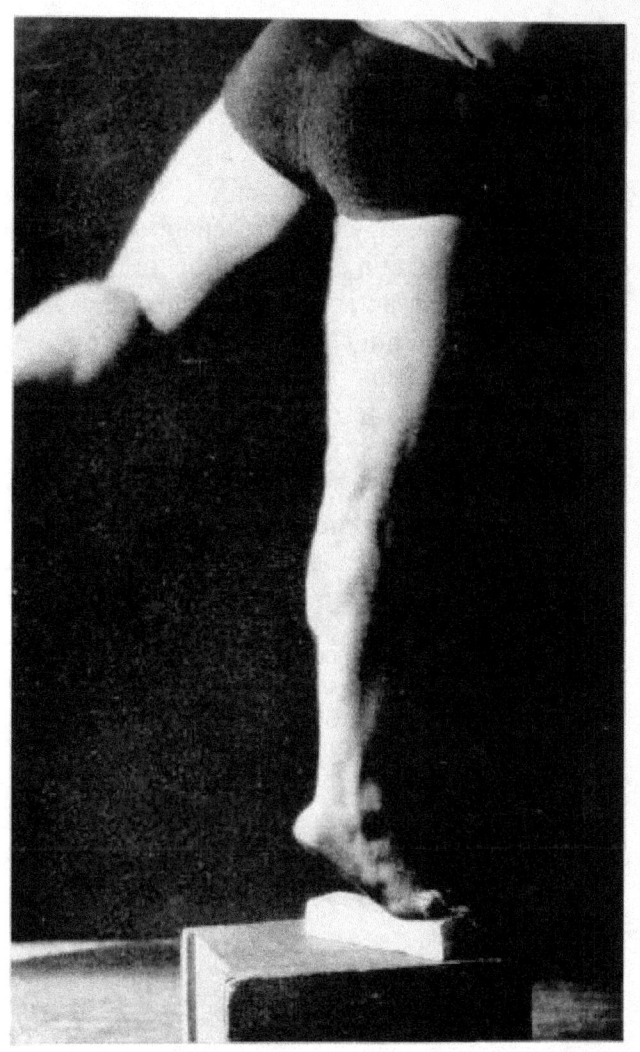

EXERCISE FOR THE CALVES

Rising up and down on one foot at a time is an excellent movement for the calf, but in order to obtain the greatest results, you should perform the movement on a block of wood or a thick book. (See chapter on the calves.)

So remember that whatever exercise you are practicing to develop the muscles of the calves, it will also help strengthen the muscles of the arches of the feet.

Exercises for the Calves

As the calves of the legs are so hard to develop, owing to constant walking, the student should not become discouraged if the progress is much slower than in other parts of his body. However, the simple rising up and down on his toes will develop the gastrocnemius muscle behind the upper calf to a certain extent. But better progress can be made if this exercise is performed on one leg at a time and the muscle is tired within twenty or twenty-five repetitions.

Still better results can be accomplished by rising up and down on the toes with the weight of a bar-bell, or a progressive exerciser that offers similar resistance. Further and quicker progress still can be made by performing this exercise against artificial resistance, with the toes resting on a book, thus giving the gastrocnemius muscle more play.

When the student eventually discovers that this last exercise is becoming too light for him, he can perform it on one leg at a time.

The shin muscle, called the tibialis anticus, really makes up the contour of the leg, when properly developed and when viewed from the front, for this muscle presents a pleasing curve to the anterior portion of the calf. It is developed by keeping the feet flat on the floor and bending the knees forward as far as possible, without raising the heels from the floor.

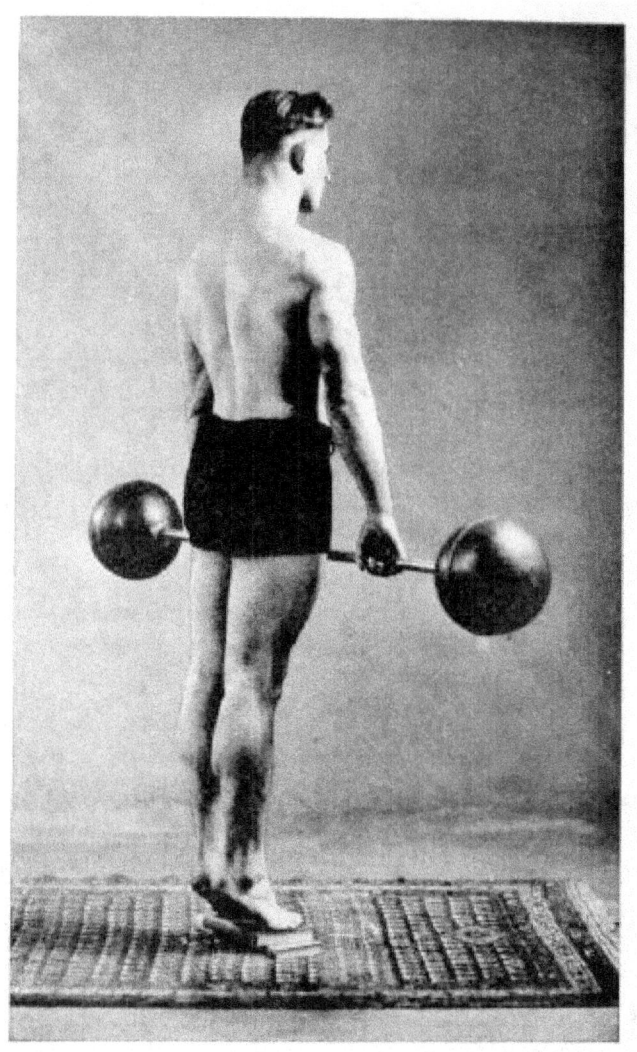

EXERCISE FOR THE CALVES

Artificial resistance is sometimes needed in calf development and in that case a bar-bell comes in handy. Rise up and down on your toes with the toes placed on a couple of books while holding a bar-bell in front of you, as shown above. (See chapter on the calves.)

If you will perform this movement with a bar-bell on your shoulder, or with someone sitting on your shoulder, you will soon observe a different appearance to your calves. Sprinting will again prove an important factor in the development of the calves, although you should limit your sprints to 100 yards at the most. Sprinting is a great developer for the calves, but endurance running is not. For, as I have said in a previous chapter, endurance runners usually have thin legs, while sprinters are well knotted up and symmetrically developed.

In order to get the most complete development of your calves, I would suggest that you secure a block of wood, or a good thick book that will raise you about four inches from the floor. Stand on this with the heels, the toes extending over the edge of the block of wood or book and touching the floor. Now raise the toes as high as you can, using the utmost strain possible. Relax and then repeat until you are tired. This is splendid for the flexor muscles on the anterior or front of the lower leg.

Then stand on the external edge of the book on your toes, and allow yourself to drop down as far as possible. Then raise slowly as far as you can, let yourself drop back, and repeat the exercise until you have a very definite ache in the muscles of the back, or posterior portion of the calf.

Now stand with the toes resting on the book, and roll the feet until the entire weight of the body rests on the outer sides of the feet. Then roll back again until the weight of the body rests on the inner sides of the feet. Repeat this exercise until the muscles in the inside and the outside of your calves feel tired.

You will find that these exercises will develop every muscle in the lower leg, and with such symmetry and uniformity that the calves will be in perfect proportion, and you will possess something that few men ever take the trouble to develop—a shapely and muscular pair of calves.

Chapter XII
Posing for Muscular Display

IN order to look your best in posing, whether it be for muscle display, or for photographic purposes, you must have the proper background and the proper lighting. For studio work, a dark red or black background is best; while a good top-light that will cast shadows under the various muscles, is always best for displaying the muscles in the picture. You should not stand directly under the top-light, but rather a little behind it.

If you will stand erect, and then while in this erect posture, bend the head forward until you see the shadow of the top of your head on the top of your chest, you will know you are in the proper light. If you stand too far back, the shadows are not so deep. If you do not use a top-light, but if instead the light should be coming from the sides or the front, it will give your muscles a flat appearance, and will not do you justice in the picture.

Posing is really an art, requiring considerable practice, if you are to acquire a posture that will show your muscles off to the best advantage. I suggest that the student practice faithfully various poses before a mirror under the proper lighting conditions, until he has found one or two, or even more, poses that are suitable for his physique.

Study the Poses of Various Athletes

It is all very well to study the various positions of others whose muscles show to great advantage in their photographs, but as no two people are built exactly alike, I do not recommend anyone to imitate another's pose unless he is sure he looks well in that position. Of course, there is the old conventional pose, which consists of folding the arms across the chest. Nearly everyone looks well in this pose, owing to the fact that the arms are photographed at angles. This makes them appear shorter and thicker than they really are. If this pose should be selected, you should make it a point to lower the shoulders when the arms are folded. Also raise the arms a little and hold the head erect, thereby showing the neck muscles and having the shoulders in a position so that they are photographed to their best advantage.

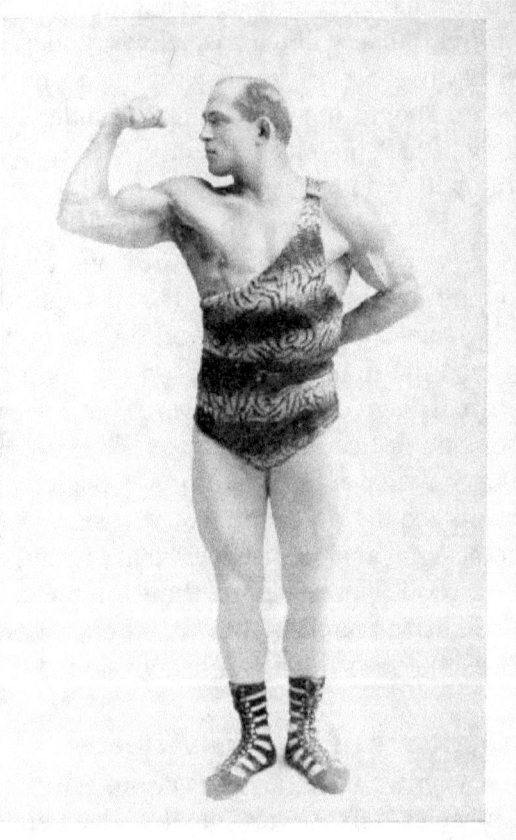

ABE BOSHES
Illustrating a standard pose assumed by many strong men. An excellent idea can be had of all-round development when an athlete assumes this posture.

If you do not lower the shoulders, the deltoids will stick up, and unless they are extremely well developed, they will look rather "pointy" in the picture, owing to the top-light.

You might possibly try a good side-light in this "folded-arms" pose and no top-light.

For this is one pose that will look well when the light comes from the sides, as it will show the pectoral development to better advantage in the shadows cast by a side-light.

No matter what light you use in this "folded-arms" pose, the forearms are going to look huge, owing to their nearness to the camera. The muscle that is placed nearest the camera naturally looks largest. I suggest that when being photographed for this "folded-arms" pose, you have your body taken from the waist up only. Do not show the legs, for you will look much stronger and heavier in a bust picture than you would in a full- length photo.

How to Show the Arms to Best Advantage

It is difficult to name the best position in which to display the arms for photographic purposes, owing to the various formations of muscles on different individuals. If you possess arms that are well muscled and knotted up, the simple front or rear flexion of the arms while held parallel to the floor will show them up to good advantage. Whether you show one arm at a time or two arms is optional with yourself, and remains to be studied, to see the effect it has upon the muscles of the shoulder and neck.

Some individuals, in flexing both arms at the height of the shoulders, have a formation of the neck muscles that causes the neck to appear thinner when the arms are placed in this position. Others have necks developed so that it makes no difference what position they hold their arms in. You should consider these facts carefully. No matter how well developed your arms are, if the muscles of your neck show to a disadvantage, you will appear to possess an awkward development in the picture.

This is another reason why I suggest that you study yourself carefully before a mirror before attempting to be photographed in a studio. For individuals whose neck development seems awkward when both arms are flexed at the height of the shoulders, I suggest that only one arm be flexed. Place the other arm behind the back, or else have the hand on the hip and turn the head to one side, in the pose of looking at your flexed biceps. By so doing, the muscles of the neck will show off to best advantage.

It takes a mighty well-developed neck to look well from all angles and under every condition. I remember years ago, when watching George Hackenschmidt, the famous wrestler, go through a series of poses, his neck did not vary one fraction of an inch when he displayed both his arms flexed at the height of his shoulder. This was because he had an especially well-developed neck.

When posing the arms, the forearm should be taken into consideration. If the wrist is turned so that the palm faces outward when the arm is flexed at the height of the shoulder, the forearm will look larger, but the biceps will appear lower and longer. But if the palm of the hand is facing the shoulder, the forearm will be a little smaller in appearance, but the biceps will be much higher.

You should never flex both arms at the same time for photographic work unless your right and left arms are exactly equal, or nearly equal, in development. If your left arm should be smaller than your right, it will be distinctly noticed in the picture, and the student of anatomy and the critic of proportions will be quick to notice this defect. If your triceps is prominently developed, it is best to show them to advantage by placing the hands behind the hips and straightening the arms. At the same time contract the latissimus dorsi muscle, pressing it against your arm. After considerable practice, this will throw out your triceps to the best possible degree. This would make a side pose.

Care should be taken regarding the lighting effect when photographing this muscle, for if the top-light should be over your chest, the triceps will not look quite as well as if the top-light were over your upper back. In other words, you will have to move around and study yourself in a mirror, which someone holds before you in front of the camera, before allowing the photographer to snap the picture. If you will expand your chest and practice certain tilts of the head while showing the triceps in this position, you will finally hit upon the right position and look your best in the picture.

Some Men Take Back and Side Poses Best

Some athletes look their best by showing part of their back, at the same time they are displaying their triceps. If the back is well knotted this will make a very good picture. If, however you have phenomenally developed pectoral muscles, it may be to your advantage to show less of the back and more of the chest when taking this pose.

While dealing with the subject of side posing, I might mention that I have seen many athletes hold their arms in various positions while turning sideways to the camera. Some even go so far as to flex one arm at the height of the shoulder and have the elbow pointed toward the camera, thereby making the arm look enormous. I do not advise this sort of posing, for any photographer or student of anatomy will realize that the arm is held near the camera, most probably for the reason that it is not sufficiently developed to show it at any other angle.

It is all very well to fool yourself, but it is pretty hard to fool everybody else. In photographic contests, judges, as a rule, do not consider the physique of anyone whose muscles are photographed sideways or on an angle—which is the result of placing a certain part of the body near the camera for the sole purpose of appearing as large as possible in that muscle or group of muscles.

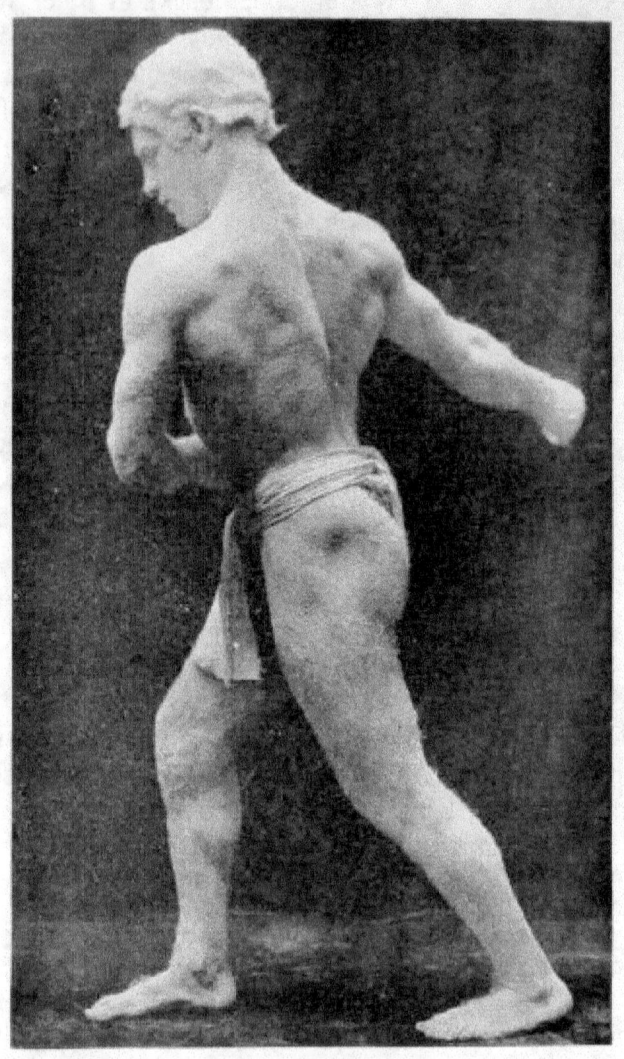

ARTHUR L. HYSON

An interesting statue pose of this well trained athlete. By smearing the body with a mixture of oxide of zinc, cold cream and glycerine, any physical culture enthusiast can obtain artistic results in photographs.

How to Photograph the Back

The back offers a very interesting display when posed under a proper light. However, the same thing that applies to the arms when flexed in a front view, also applies to the arms when flexed in a rear view. Unless your arms are equally developed, do not attempt to show both arms together, but show one at a time, holding the other arm behind your back. While being photographed in this position, you should flex the arm that is held behind your back just as thoroughly as you flex the arm that you are endeavoring to show.

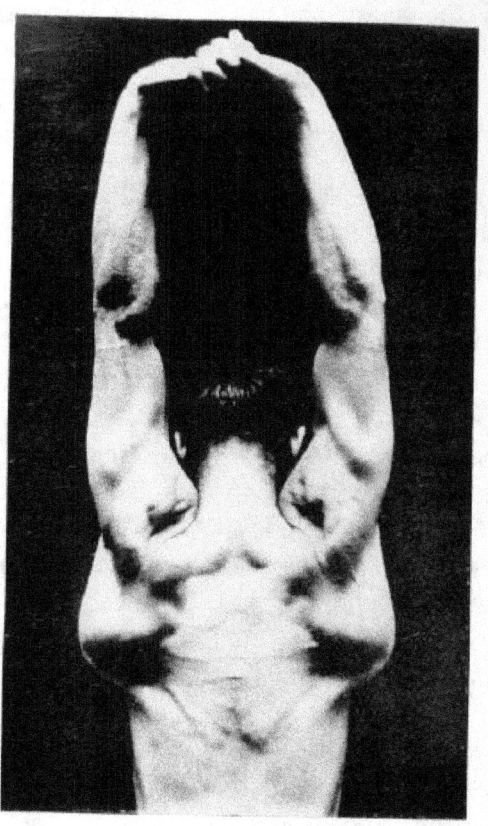

EARLE LIEDERMAN
Showing control of the upper back muscles. This photograph was taken in 1907, when the author first acquired some of his muscles.

I also advise you to inhale as deeply as possible and contract the latissimus dorsi muscles to their limit. At the same time, turn the head slightly, so that the profile of your face will show yourself looking at your flexed biceps. If your arms are equally developed, it is all very well to show both together, but the neck should again be taken into consideration.

The neck, in this instance, differs from the neck as photographed in the front view, for only a slight change is noted when photographing the neck from the rear view, even though the arms are held at the height of the shoulders. However, the chin should be kept in and the head thrown slightly backwards, if you desire your neck to have a straight appearance. In this pose, however, the neck will not look quite as large as it will if you bend your head forward.

By bending the head forward, the head naturally is further away from the camera. The top of your head will therefore look smaller, making your neck look bigger than if you bent your neck backward, thus placing the top of the head a little nearer the camera, and making the head appear larger. The larger your head appears in a photograph, the smaller you yourself will look, and vice versa.

Another interesting back pose that looks well in a picture under the proper lighting is the expansion of the scapulas or shoulder blades. While contracting the teres major muscle and causing this muscle to pull the scapula to its extreme limit, hold the hands overhead, keeping the arms stiff. Either clasp one hand with the other, or else interlace the fingers. Now while raising the shoulders very slightly, pull apart vigorously with your hands. After considerable practice, you will be able to observe two prominent lumps protruding at each side of the upper back, when viewed from the front, and when viewed from the rear by the camera, it will show an interesting muscular display, produced by the aid of the scapula, or shoulder blade.

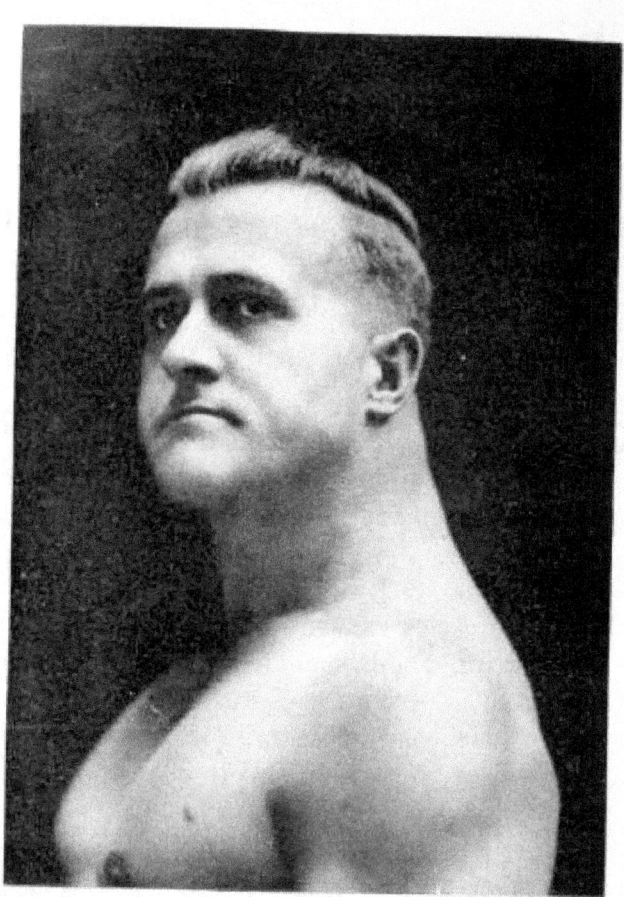

EARLE LIEDERMAN

As he is today. Showing development of the neck and height of normal chest.

In photographing the muscles of the back, the student must have a top-light to produce the best effect, for a wonderful display can be had if the proper lighting and background are used and the proper pose assumed.

How to Place the Camera Lens

If the camera lens is placed on a level with your face, your head will appear larger and your legs will appear smaller, whereas if the camera lens is placed about the height of your waist, your torso and legs will appear in their natural proportions and your head will be somewhat smaller, thus causing an optical illusion in your photograph.

On the other hand, if the lens of the camera is placed at the height of your waist, your biceps will not look as large as they will if the lens of the camera is pointed at the height of your arms. This is especially noticed when being photographed from rear view, with the arms flexed at the height of your shoulders.

To give you a clear idea of this optical illusion, if you ever have had the opportunity of looking down from a platform at some athlete, you will observe that he looks much smaller, looking down at him, than if he were on the platform and you looked up at him.

How to Display the Neck Muscles

The neck muscles can be thrown out to a remarkable degree by drawing both shoulders forward. Contract the chest and reach downward as far as possible, at the same time bending the head backwards. This, however, is an awkward pose for photographic work and I do not suggest any student adopting it. I simply mention it as one of the series of poses that can be put in your routine whenever the occasion warrants it.

The neck can also be shown in this manner from the rear. After practice, the student will be able to throw out his neck without reaching downward and by holding his arms sideways at the height of the shoulders, thereby giving an interesting display of the trapezius muscle as well.

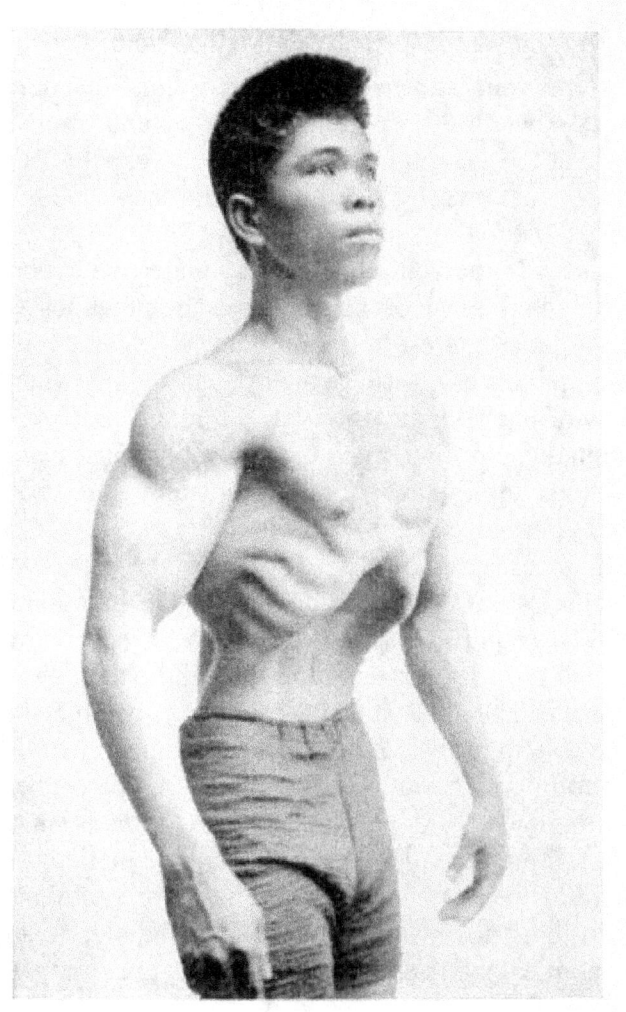

SIMON JAVIERTO

Displaying phenomenal abdominal control. This abdominal cavity is sucked in by complete exhalation of all air from the lungs—the abdominal wall then filling up the vacuum.

Photographing the Abdominal Muscles

The abdominal region offers one of the most interesting studies in the way of muscular posing. The most simple abdominal contraction consists of stooping slightly forward and pressing upon the thighs with the hands, giving a washboard effect to the front of the abdomen. A little more difficult pose is to display the control of the abdominal cavity. In your endeavors to secure this diaphragmatic control, expel all the air from your lungs, and bend slightly forward at the same time. When the air is expelled, draw in the abdominal muscles until they fill up the vacuum caused by the exhalation of your diaphragm.

This will give you a deep cavity under the rib box and even though it is one of the frequent abdominal poses, yet it is one of great interest to the spectator. The camera will not photograph this as clearly as the eye can see it, owing to the shadow of the rib box. However, if you desire to show this abdominal control in a picture, I suggest you use side-lights as well as top-lights in order to display the abdominal cavity to best advantage.

Still another interesting display of the rectus abdominus muscles consists of single and double isolation of this group. To acquire this, the air must be expelled from the lungs and a cavity formed under the rib box, as previously mentioned. Then the student, after considerable practice, will be able to throw out one side of his abdominal muscles by a strong pressure of the forearm on the top of the thigh, in the region of the sartorius muscle. In addition to this downward pressure, the pressure should be inclined slightly outward as well. By pressing both hands on each inner side of the thighs downward and outward, double isolation of the abdominal wall can be obtained. This undoubtedly gives the most interesting display of the contraction of the abdominal muscles for photographic purposes. In this case, no side-light is needed, for a side-light would be superfluous and spoil the effect of this muscular display.

The student should not be discouraged if he is unable to acquire this abdominal isolation during the first month of his attempts, but if diligent practice is pursued, success will eventually come.

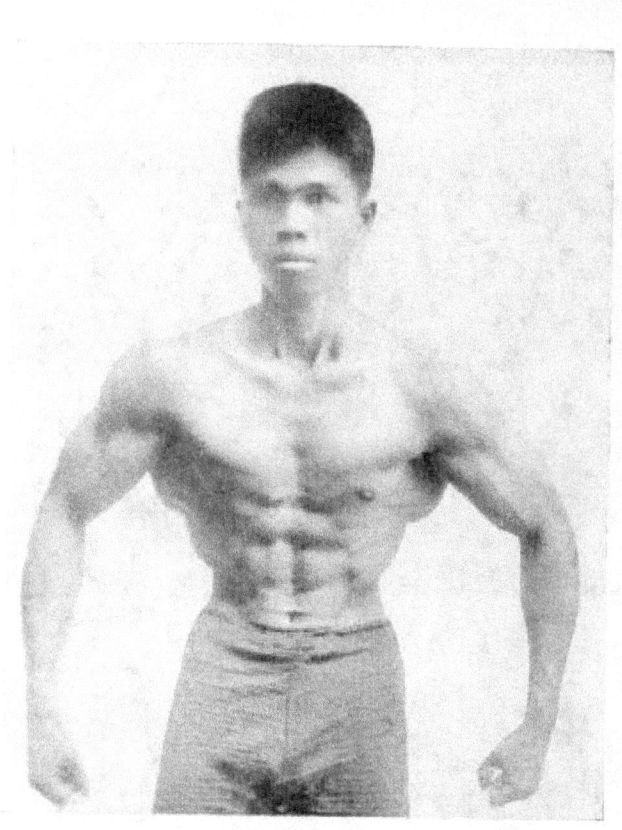

SIMON JAVIERTO

Showing isolation of the abdominal muscles. This control is accomplished by complete exhalation of all air from the lungs, drawing in the abdominal wall to fill the vacuum, and then, by bending slightly forward, contracting the rectus abdominus muscles.

To Display the Muscles of the Thighs and Calves

The muscles of the thighs are best displayed by turning the toes outward, in order to show the curve of the quadriceps extensor muscles. If, however, you possess thighs that are exceptionally developed in the extensor femoris muscle, or the outside of the legs, perhaps a plain front view of the thighs would suit your case better. In that case, the toes should be pointed forward. You must study this yourself, and see from what angle your legs will photograph best.

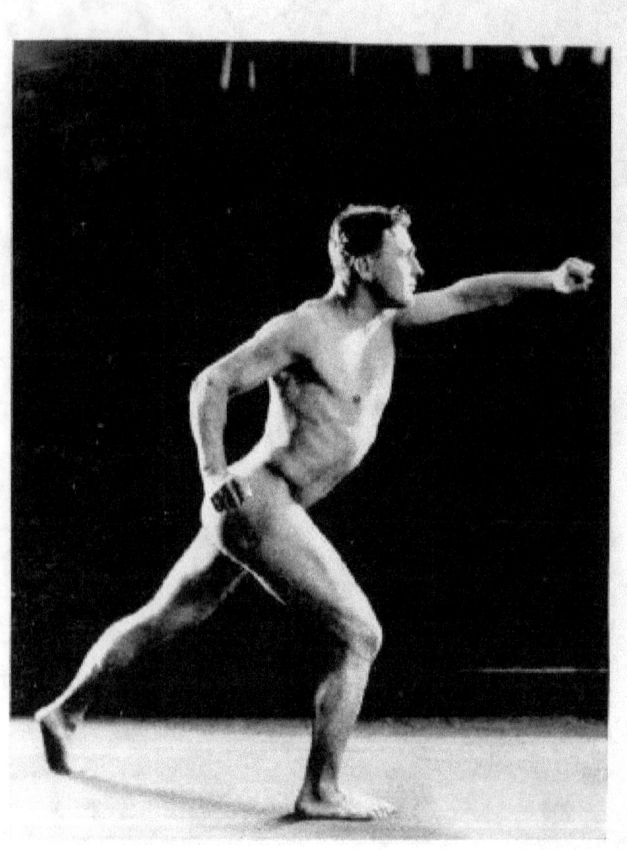

JESSE M. GEHMAN
An athlete of the lighter type whose well balanced proportions add greatly to the action in his pose.

If the calves of your legs are not developed to quite as satisfactory proportions as the rest of your physique, I suggest that you wear sandals that will come half way up your legs, thereby eliminating a long, slim ankle. If, however, you are short of stature and your legs and ankles are well proportioned, ordinary gymnasium shoes, or even no shoes at all, will undoubtedly be best suited for your purpose.

Care should be taken as to what costume to wear when posing for a picture. I suggest that the student wear a pair of ordinary black bathing trunks and roll these trunks well up toward the crotch. Also roll the top part down about two inches below the navel. This gives you the opportunity of displaying your thighs and abdominal muscles to their best advantage.

If the tights extend above the navel or to the middle of the thigh, it will detract greatly from your appearance and make you look like an amateur. I recommend these trunks as better than anything else to wear while posing, for they will photograph much better than any other material or costume that you may use.

Many professional athletes wear leopard skins and sandals. This costume gives them a decidedly professional and finished appearance, but to my mind, it draws the attention away from the muscles, which should be the important part of the picture. Still others wear wrist bands which give an impression of stronger arms than they really have, but these also detract from muscular display and make the arms appear shorter. There is no need for anyone to adopt artificial means in order to display the muscles to the best advantage. If you are lacking in muscular display in any part of your body, my best advice to you is to exercise more diligently on this defective part, thereby developing it and satisfying your desires, and do not try to get by on a fake. For the one person in all this world whom you do not want to fake, and whom it would never pay you to fool, is yourself.

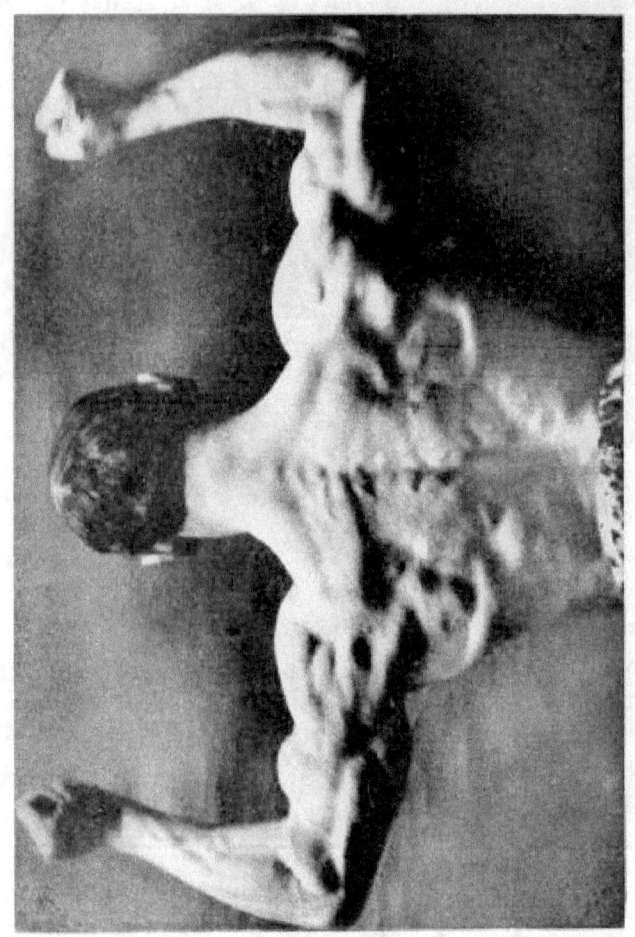

F. ROLLON

An exceptionally fine example of back development. It shows the interesting formation in which the back muscles can be displayed.

****

AFTER you have attained the results you desire, it is a very simple matter to merely perform light work every day in order to keep in shape. At that time you do not have to continually strive for progress unless you want to, but all this time you are striving for your maximum measurements you are ever increasing your strength and energy, thus building up your internal organs and acquiring a physique that will carry you through the rest of your life—a strong, healthy, robust man.

If, by chance, any reader of this book should never have tried any systematic exercise, to him I say, everything awaits you, and if you will only put forth your honest endeavors for three months' time, not only will you look and act like an altogether new person, but you will be so enthusiastic over your progress that you will gladly retain your enthusiasm for another nine months until you have strength and development far above the average individual, and you will never again know or be bothered with the numerous ailments that continually affect the average non physical culturist.

Isn't this worth striving for?

I want to pass a final little thought to you. No matter what your age may be, the best time to form good resolutions is right now when you are younger than you will ever again be in your life.

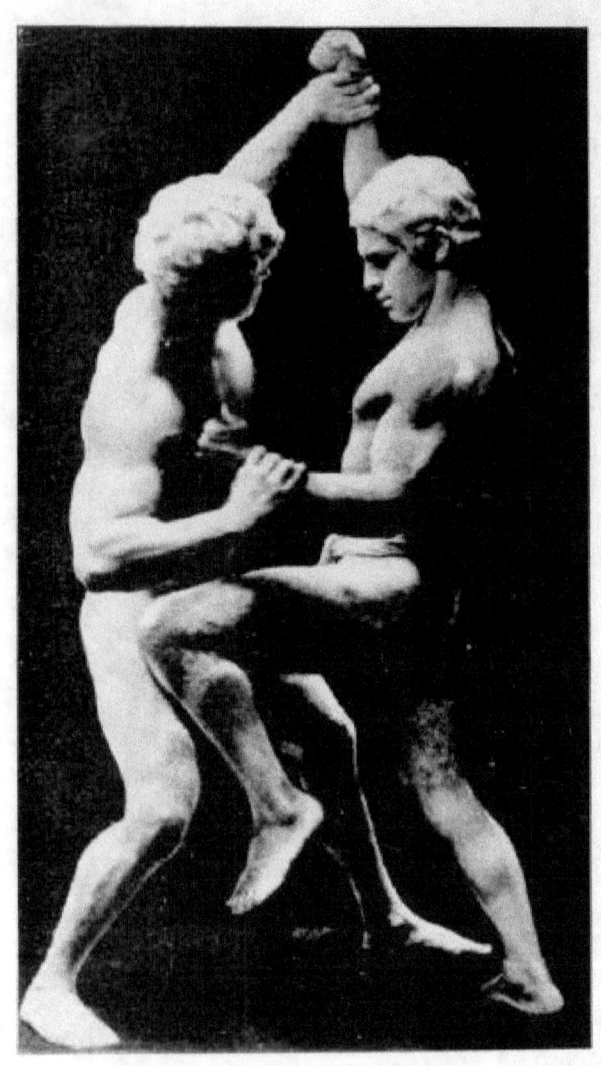

Earle Liederman (left) and Arthur Hyson (right) in an artistic statue pose.